Download Your Included Ebook Today!

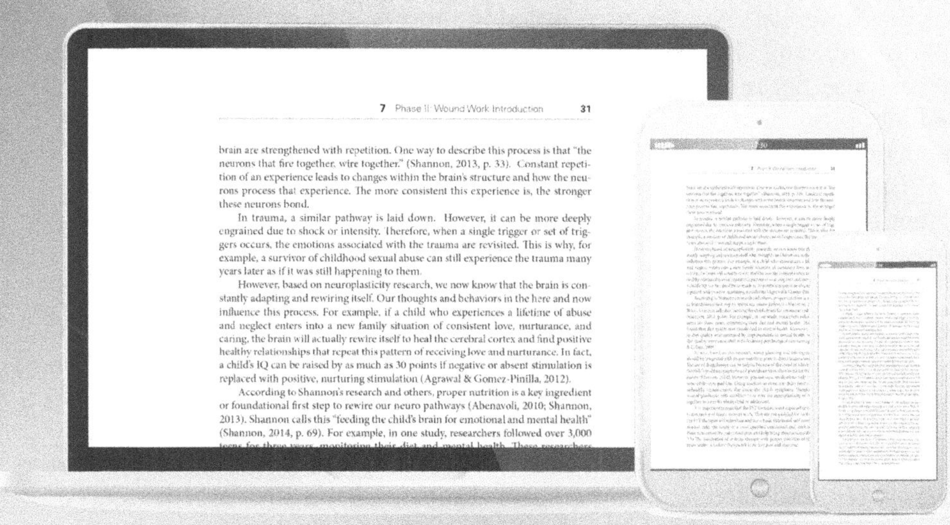

Your print purchase of *Academic Leadership in Nursing: Effective Strategies for Aspiring Faculty and Leaders* **includes an ebook download** to the device of your choice—increasing accessibility, portability, and searchability!

Download your ebook today at:
http://spubonline.com/faculty
and enter the access code below:

1WHGG55S8

SPC

Leslie Neal-Boylan, PhD, RN, APRN, FAAN, is the associate dean and professor of nursing at the Massachusetts General Hospital (MGH) Institute of Health Professions, the educational arm of the MGH. She was formerly the dean of nursing at University of Wisconsin–Oshkosh in Oshkosh, Wisconsin. She is a certified family nurse practitioner, a fellow of the American Academy of Nursing, and is also certified in rehabilitation nursing. Dr. Neal-Boylan's scholarship focuses on the nursing workforce; her most recent work concerns nurses with disabilities. She is widely published, having written more than 100 peer-reviewed articles and nine books, three of which have won the coveted *American Journal of Nursing* Book of the Year award. She is also a winner of the Virginia Henderson Excellence in Research award and serves on several nursing organizations, including Sigma Theta Tau, and editorial boards.

Sharron E. Guillett, PhD, RN, is a retired campus president of Chamberlain University, Chamberlain College of Nursing, Downers Grove, Illinois. Prior to that, she served as a campus dean for Stratford University, Falls Church, Virginia, and prior to that was chair of the BSN program at Marymount University, Arlington, Virginia, where she was a tenured faculty member, and director of the RN–BSN program. She has held a number of leadership positions over her 40-year career in healthcare, educational, research, and clinical settings. She has managed the creation and accreditation of nursing programs, and is experienced in the administration of research grant programs as well as direct healthcare delivery. She has authored a book on chronic care, and has written numerous peer-reviewed journal articles on a variety of topics. Dr. Guillett is a long-standing member of Sigma Theta Tau.

Sharon Chappy, PhD, RN, CNOR, currently is dean and professor at the School of Nursing at Concordia University, Wisconsin. She previously served in various leadership roles at the University of Wisconsin–Oshkosh. Her research areas include nursing education, perioperative nursing, evidence-based practice issues, and patients with cancer and their perceptions of care. She has published in peer-reviewed journals on all of these areas. Dr. Chappy has been research editor of the *AORN Journal* and is an active member of the Association of periOperative Registered Nurses (AORN), serving on various national committees and jointly authoring documents guiding perioperative nursing practice. She is a member of the Wisconsin Nurses Association, the American Nurses Association, and the Phi Beta Chapter of Sigma Theta Tau.

ACADEMIC LEADERSHIP IN NURSING

Effective Strategies for Aspiring Faculty and Leaders

Leslie Neal-Boylan, PhD, RN, APRN, FAAN

Sharron E. Guillett, PhD, RN

Sharon Chappy, PhD, RN, CNOR

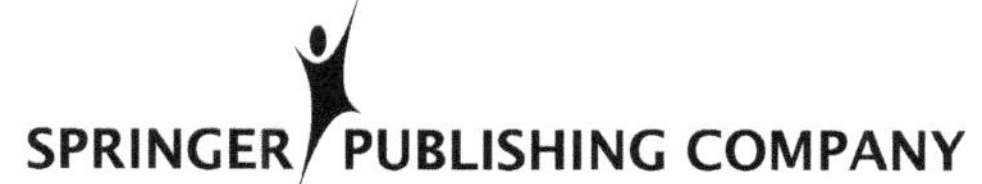

SPRINGER PUBLISHING COMPANY

Springer Publishing Company, LLC
11 West 42nd Street
New York, NY 10036
www.springerpub.com

Acquisitions Editor: Joseph Morita
Compositor: diacriTech, Chennai

ISBN: 978-0-8261-3452-3
ebook ISBN: 978-0-8261-3453-0

18 19 20 21 22 / 5 4 3 2 1

The author and the publisher of this Work have made every effort to use sources believed to be reliable to provide information that is accurate and compatible with the standards generally accepted at the time of publication. Because medical science is continually advancing, our knowledge base continues to expand. Therefore, as new information becomes available, changes in procedures become necessary. We recommend that the reader always consult current research and specific institutional policies before performing any clinical procedure. The author and publisher shall not be liable for any special, consequential, or exemplary damages resulting, in whole or in part, from the readers' use of, or reliance on, the information contained in this book. The publisher has no responsibility for the persistence or accuracy of URLs for external or third-party Internet websites referred to in this publication and does not guarantee that any content on such websites is, or will remain, accurate or appropriate.

Library of Congress Cataloging-in-Publication Data
Names: Neal-Boylan, Leslie, author. | Guillett, Sharron E., author. | Chappy,
  Sharon, author.
Title: Academic leadership in nursing : effective strategies for aspiring
  faculty and leaders / Leslie Neal-Boylan, Sharron Guillett, Sharon Chappy.
Description: New York, NY : Springer Publishing Company, LLC, [2018] |
  Includes bibliographical references and index.
Identifiers: LCCN 2017056808 | ISBN 9780826134523 | ISBN 9780826134530 (ebook)
Subjects: | MESH: Faculty, Nursing-standards | Leadership | Schools, Nursing
Classification: LCC RT90 | NLM WY 105 | DDC 610.73071/1—dc23 LC record available at
https://lccn.loc.gov/2017056808

CONTENTS

PREFACE

We decided to write this book to share what we have learned and wish we had known when we became academic leaders. Other books on academic leadership may not be specific to nursing and we could find none that compared the experiences of nursing faculty or academic leaders among public, private, and for-profit or proprietary institutions. Although there are certainly similarities, there are also key differences. We each walked into our positions without knowing or understanding these differences, but we all agree that, had we known, the information would have had a significant impact on our decisions and choices. There are also misconceptions and myths about each of these types of organizations.

Like so much else about faculty and academic leadership positions, there is only so much one can research beforehand. Much of what we need to know, such as the culture of an organization, must be experienced. We thought that sharing details about the differences and similarities across public, private, and for-profit institutions specific to nursing education would enlighten and inform current and future faculty and academic leaders to enable you to make decisions about your academic career. Although we recognize that readers may work in or seek to work in schools, departments, or colleges of nursing, for simplicity we chose to use the phrase "school of nursing," or SON, to represent all of these.

The Introduction is a "conversation" among the authors regarding why it is important to know how public, private, and for-profit educational organizations operate and why nurse educators and academic leaders should take the time to learn this information.

Chapter 1 explains the structures of these organizations. Chapter 2 offers concrete suggestions and tips for successfully applying for a faculty position in each of these organizations, whereas Chapter 3 does the same for seeking an academic leadership position. Chapter 4 explains and discusses the nuances of fund-raising and advancement. Recruiting qualified and diverse faculty and staff is challenging and processes vary depending on the type of institution; so recruitment is discussed in Chapter 5. Marketing and public relations are increasingly important in both faculty and leadership positions. Chapter 6 explores these topics. In nursing education, we are all challenged by acquiring and developing clinical partnerships. The authors offer tried-and-true suggestions in Chapter 7. Chapter 8 discusses budgeting and the allocation of resources. Academic leaders especially must be knowledgeable in these areas. Chapter 9 discusses maintaining nursing education standards via accreditation processes and board of nursing approval. Each author has extensive experience with this and is eager to share lessons learned. Chapter 10 explores how to encourage faculty and staff to think innovatively and describes similarities and differences pertaining to international study among the three types of institutions. Finally, the Conclusion (Chapter 11) is a "conversation" among the authors, who share their visions for the future in public, private, and for-profit schools of nursing.

Each chapter is divided into sections, offering public, for-profit, and private university perspectives. However, in some topic areas, content may overlap; readers are encouraged to read each chapter in its entirety or risk missing valuable information that may apply to all three types of universities.

Leslie Neal-Boylan
Sharron E. Guillett
Sharon Chappy

ACKNOWLEDGMENTS

Many thanks to my very supportive husband, Dr. Kevin M. Boylan, and to nurse educators everywhere. Regardless of the type of school in which we work, we all work very hard to ensure the success of our students and to preserve the quality of our most esteemed profession.

Leslie Neal-Boylan

I would like to thank my husband, Warren, and my children, Brian, Alexis, and Amanda, for their consistent encouragement. I would also like to thank my coauthors for their commitment, integrity, and generosity in this endeavor.

Sharron E. Guillett

Thank you to my husband, Michael, and our children, Abby and Adam, for their unending support and amazing ability to keep me laughing. Also thank you to the countless mentors, peers, and colleagues who have provided me wisdom and experiences that contributed to my personal and professional journey through life.

Sharon Chappy

INTRODUCTION: A CONVERSATION WITH DRS. NEAL-BOYLAN, GUILLETT, AND CHAPPY

Why is it important for faculty and prospective or current academic nurse leaders to compare public, private, and for-profit nursing programs?

Dr. Guillett: There are a number of reasons why it is important to understand the varying organizational structures underpinning nursing education. Ultimately, we are all concerned about the quality of nursing education across programs, states, and countries. Nursing, as a profession, has a commitment, a contract with society, to provide the best care possible to all. Faculty and administrators have great responsibility for delivering on this commitment. It is up to this group of individuals to ensure that *all* educational programs produce high-quality graduates. We need to understand that there is more than one pathway to that goal and move away from the dichotomous worldview that holds if one type of program is good all others must be bad, when in fact they are just different. "Goodness," or quality standards, can and are met in each organizational structure and yet we devalue educational experiences different from our own. Remember the way in which diploma grads were marginalized when the bachelor of science in nursing (BSN) became entry to the profession? When we understand what each program offers and where each program can improve, we help students, faculty, and administrators make better decisions and, on a larger scale, improve outcomes for all of society.

Dr. Neal-Boylan: I agree that it is important to recognize that each type of organizational structure makes some unique contributions to nursing education. When we look for a faculty or academic leadership position, there is a lot we can research beforehand, such as board pass rates and the programs and services provided to students. However, we cannot really understand the culture within the organization or school of nursing (SON) until we experience it. A comprehensive understanding of how organizational structure and processes differ among public, private, and for-profit institutions can better prepare prospective faculty and academic leaders before they agree to work for an organization. Not only will this information impress interviewers because the reader has done her or his homework, but the information can help nurse educators make informed choices about the place they would like to work. Knowing how to teach and work with students and faculty is really not enough. There are so many other variables that impact a satisfying and successful experience as a member of the faculty or in a position of leadership. The more one knows before starting in any position, the better.

Dr. Chappy: When nursing faculty and administrators are looking for new professional opportunities, they may often mistakenly look at salary, geographic location, and even school reputation as primary motivators for a change. Although these variables are very important in enticing someone to leave a current job and move into a new position, there are so many other factors that are influential in achieving professional satisfaction. The culture and organizational structure of an organization are two critical variables. When educators move from "what they know" to "something different" it can be a real shock if they are not adequately prepared for the realities of the unique attributes of public, private, and for-profit nursing programs. Personal values must be aligned with the organizational culture or true professional contentment cannot be achieved. Studying the nuances of how public, private, and for-profit organizations work before blindly moving into an organization will ensure a good fit and overall job satisfaction.

What inspired you to write this book?

Dr. Guillett: I received my doctoral degree from a large public institution where I was privileged to work closely with faculty who were well known nationally. These faculty included me in their publications (books and articles), research, and committee work. I observed firsthand what the organizational structure supported and prevented. I actually applied for a faculty position but was told, as were others of my class, that the school did not hire its own grads. Really? I also learned how powerful the dean was and how careful you had to be when you were around her. The hierarchy of academe is an "old boy/old girl" network not to be underestimated. Acceptance and advancement were not always awarded on the basis of merit but on currying favor. Some years later, once I had established myself in the field as an educator, researcher, and author, and there was a new dean at the helm, I once again inquired about a faculty position. This time, I was not even granted an interview because I did not have research money to bring with me to supplement my income.

I spent over 10 years teaching at a private Catholic school where I became a tenured professor and truly grew as a professional. I became the director of the undergraduate program and president of the faculty council. I learned about the regulatory aspects of the program and the accreditation process at both the program and university levels. I enjoyed the position immensely. But, when I was offered an opportunity to open a nursing program (something I was very interested in doing) at a small for-profit school with a six-figure salary (much more than I was currently making), I accepted. I did not know how different leading and teaching at a for-profit school would be. I had no idea how being associated with a for-profit school would impact opportunities for both my program and me. Had I fully understood the differences in philosophy, priorities, and organizational structure, I doubt I would have made the move. It turned out not only to be a good move, but an extremely rewarding one. Nursing programs in the for-profit sector are of the highest quality and meet all of the state and accreditation requirements of traditional programs. The challenges are different and are real. Balancing the need to meet the budget and maintain quality is an ongoing struggle. Helping people in business understand and value nursing's paradigm, code of ethics, and commitment to quality can be a challenge. But the opportunity to change lives is very real. The students who come to for-profits are usually making great personal sacrifices to be there. Many are disadvantaged socio-economically. Most are seeking a better way of life for themselves and their families.

Providing the pathway to a new and better life is tremendously fulfilling and while this sense of accomplishment can be found in all educational settings, it is up close and personal in the for-profit sector. Because of the flat organizational structure, you know your students really well. Most for-profits understand the importance of having a relationship with the students and promote it and support it financially. Successful programs have faculty/student mentoring programs that start at admission. My current school follows and stays connected to students after graduation and supports them right up to licensure. We, all nursing educators, are concerned about pass rates. However, in my experience, for-profits take a more individualized approach to address that concern.

So, my purpose in writing this book is to share what I know about the for-profit sector from an insider's view of programs offered in both family-owned and publicly traded organizations and how they compare with traditional programs in which I also have considerable experience. For-profits are different; that does not make them less desirable. I want to share that fact with the world. For-profits are valuable; the faculty and staff are high-quality practitioners and scholars who do research and publish and practice at the bedside. They work with the National League for Nursing (NLN) and American Nurses Association (ANA) and some have chapters with Sigma Theta Tau International (STTI). Graduates of for-profits work in all healthcare arenas and go on to pursue advanced degrees. The for-profit sector is focused on business; the business happens to be education. This is not a good fit for everyone. I hope that the information in this book will help you decide whether it is a good fit for you.

Dr. Neal-Boylan: I was inspired to write this book because I have good friends and colleagues who work as nurse educators and academic leaders in public, private, and for-profit institutions. We have shared our concerns, experiences, successes, and failures. Having taught and worked in private and public universities, large and small, I was already aware of those inherent differences. I knew my colleagues in for-profit schools were often unfairly maligned. I confess that I had serious misconceptions about for-profit programs. I realized that it was unfair to judge other programs without understanding their reality. I also thought that if I could benefit from this knowledge, then other nurses could too. The information in this book is vital to anyone considering a faculty or academic leadership role in nursing or who is considering moving to a different type of institution. I have learned a lot from my coauthors and I am certain you will, too.

Dr. Chappy: I had several professional mentors. Two who have been the most influential are Professor Emerita Ellen K. Murphy from the University of Wisconsin–Milwaukee, and former dean Rosemary Smith from the University of Wisconsin–Oshkosh. Professor Murphy mentored me in my earlier research and teaching career. She provided me with opportunities for rigorous scholarship and for service opportunities at a national level. I made the most of every one of those opportunities and people began to notice my work. Success in one opportunity led to more opportunities. I was always looking! I was never afraid to work hard and I was never afraid to fail, but mostly I succeeded at what I did.

Dr. Rosemary Smith gave me professional and other leadership opportunities at the public university in which I worked for 17 years. She supported me as I advanced in rank and as I moved into various administrative roles. For several years, she told me I was "ready to be a dean" and she supported me in attending conferences and seminars that would build my leadership skills and abilities, and would help to fill my "dean toolbox." I began looking for dean opportunities; there were so many out there that the possibilities were almost endless. She coached me, gave advice, and wrote letters of reference. She was retiring soon, but I decided I was ready and that my timeline could not wait for her to retire, so I looked outside my organization. I looked to a private school. I was fortunate to have been offered the first job as dean for which I interviewed. I was a finalist for another job but withdrew before the on-campus interview because when I interviewed for my current job, I knew that I desperately wanted it and felt confident that it would be offered to me. I was ready to make the move from a public to a private school.

Even though I had done my homework, nothing prepared me fully for the change, not only to a private school, but also to move into the role of dean. The differences in public, private, and for-profit schools are not bad or good . . . but there are many differences. I never regretted my move; it truly was one of the best professional decisions I have ever made. I kept notes from the very beginning of my deanship about "things I wish I had known." Sometimes, I made mistakes just because I did not know the rules. Sometimes, I had difficulty understanding the culture. When the opportunity came up to contribute to this book, it was the perfect time to pull out all my notes and share them with you. I hope that by giving you my "lessons learned," it will better prepare any of you who might be looking to move into a private organization.

Why are the topics addressed in this book particularly important to faculty and prospective or current academic leaders?

Dr. Guillett: Most of us start a job thinking we will try it out for a couple of years and, before you know it, 5 years have gone by during which time we either positioned ourselves well for what comes next or we find ourselves "stuck." The information presented here is extremely important in ensuring the former. It is a deep dive into the milieu of the educational workplace and answers questions you probably did not think to ask. Is research one of your long-term goals? Are you trying to break into a leadership role or being offered an opportunity in a sector that is different from where you currently practice? Knowing what to look for and what to ask about can help you make the best decision possible.

Dr. Neal-Boylan: I fell into my first academic leadership position in a private Catholic school where I had been teaching; then followed leadership positions in public and private programs. I did not know about any of the nuances described in this book until I had already started in these positions. Frequently, as faculty we are so absorbed in all of our work teaching, practicing, conducting research, and sitting on committees and boards that we do not get the opportunity to really learn how the organization for which we work really operates and how its operation impacts the direction and operations of the SON. In leadership roles, such as a director or chair, we are exposed to more of this information. However, as dean, one is responsible and accountable for SON operations and must have a detailed understanding of how the university works and how its processes impact our operations. Developing this understanding *before* you apply for a faculty or leadership position can save you a lot of future questions and anxiety and give you peace of mind that you are entering into a position with fewer secrets to discover.

Dr. Chappy: When I was offered my first dean position, which I now hold, I looked for books and articles on becoming a dean. I found only two that were relevant: *The Growth and Development of Nurse Leaders*, by Angela McBride, and *Nursing Leadership from the Outside In*, edited by Greer Glazer and Joyce Fitzpatrick. I read them both within a day or two, but wanted more! I had so many questions and I wanted to be as best prepared as I could, but there just was nothing more out there. So this book provides a comprehensive resource for potential faculty and those looking to become administrative leaders to use in weighing decisions and in informing choices. When we got together to decide topics for each chapter, it was amazing how all three coauthors targeted the same topics as the most important ones for which to share information.

What specific experience did you bring to the dean role that has helped make you a successful academic leader?

Dr. Guillett: I have held leadership roles in all aspects of my life, personal and professional. Each of these has helped me understand the diverse ways that people respond to leadership styles, communication styles, carry out assigned activities, and so forth. Working in service-focused organizations, such as Easter Seals and the National Association of Children's Hospitals and Related Institutions (NACHRI), helped me see the bigger picture and how to accomplish big goals (like healthcare reform) incrementally through collaboration. I think the experiences that have helped me the most have been the opportunities to collaborate with other leaders both in nursing and other disciplines on committees, boards, and workshops, and at national conferences. I learned much through these encounters, such as how to listen, negotiate, manage conflict, build consensus, and leverage partnerships.

Dr. Neal-Boylan: I have always maintained a clinical practice throughout my academic career and I think this has helped me in the role of dean. Not only has that experience given me credibility with students and faculty, but I think it has kept me current regarding what students need to know to work safely and successfully as nurses.

My long experience as faculty and later as a cochair of an associate degree program, chair of a graduate program, and associate dean also prepared me to be a dean. The transition from the faculty role to the administrative role, especially to the associate dean or dean roles, is significant. There are so many details to learn and consider, personnel issues to confront and help resolve, and decisions to weigh in on, that experience as a director or chair is extremely helpful to help educate oneself to be an administrator. As faculty, I had no idea what the dean was doing or was expected to do and I had little time to concern myself with what she or he was doing. I was simply grateful that I had a competent leader. Many faculty think they know what a dean does or is required to do or know, but faculty are not privy, despite transparency and shared governance, to everything that happens within a university on a daily basis. My scholarly work also prepared me to be a dean because I was able to lead and mentor faculty in their scholarly work. I was able to say, "If I can do it, you can do it" and it is important that leaders model the behavior they expect from others.

Dr. Chappy: Like Dr. Neal-Boylan, I continued to practice as a perioperative nurse for most of my academic career, until about 5 years ago. As Dr. Neal-Boylan noted, this helped me to truly understand what student nurses needed to know to be successful registered nurses and my experiences allowed me to "live" the very rapid changes within healthcare that my nonpracticing colleagues often did not see. As a qualitative researcher, I always want to be deeply involved with people and know the "breadth and depth" of a situation. That has helped me listen and understand others better. I have always been a firm believer in the crucial conversations foundation: Say what you mean; do not sugarcoat or give mixed messages or the true meaning may not be conveyed. I am direct and honest. That can be unappealing to some, but most appreciate knowing my meaning and my message clearly. My experiences with research and publishing have honed my writing skills. Written messages can be very powerful and can reach wide audiences. My goal has always been to influence the profession of nursing in a positive way, and I think I have accomplished that.

What is the charge/mission for the university?

Dr. Guillett: Mission statements reflect goals, not purposes. Therefore, while the purpose of any for-profit enterprise is to make money, the mission will address the goal of educating and preparing students for a better life. Universities that have many programs will have broad mission statements, whereas colleges that offer only nursing will have very specific mission statements that speak to the nursing graduate in particular.

Dr. Neal-Boylan: The ultimate mission of a public university is to educate the public and make higher education accessible and affordable so that everyone has the opportunity to obtain a college education. Each public institution has its own distinct mission and vision statements and its strategic plans will reflect the primary goals for the institution. Public universities often list their mission and/or that of the wider system within which they function, if applicable.

Dr. Chappy: The missions of private universities are as unique as their foundational tenets. However, those foundational tenets pervade the mission to educate those students who choose to attend the university and to prepare students for specific roles in life that may include service, global citizenship, or a life devoted to their faith.

REFERENCES

McBride, A. (2011). *The growth and development of nurse leaders*. New York, NY: Springer Publishing.

Glazer, G., & Fitzpatrick, J. (Eds.). (2013). *Nursing leadership from the outside in*. New York, NY: Springer Publishing.

CHAPTER 1

NAVIGATING ORGANIZATIONAL STRUCTURES AND PROCESSES

Public, for-profit, and private schools of nursing (SON) operate differently and have different formal and informal organizational structures. Both faculty and administrators or aspiring administrators should understand and at least be aware of these differences and any similarities, to make an informed choice among SON. The organizational structures of both the university and the SON can shed light on the layers of approvals, bureaucracy, and requirements with which faculty and, to a greater extent, administrators have to contend in their daily work.

■ THE PUBLIC UNIVERSITY PERSPECTIVE

Public universities and colleges may stand alone or may be governed by a system that binds all of the universities and includes system-wide policies. Consequently, the public university may have its own board of trustees or a system-wide board—a Board of Regents or Board of Trustees—that governs the university. In addition, public universities tend to have senates or councils, such as a faculty senate, that make recommendations to university leadership.

> In public institutions these core organizational entities collaborate with such external authorities as state and federal political leaders, community organizations, and members of the public, as well as business interests and philanthropic foundations. These external organizations routinely interact with and shape the policies and procedures of the university's internal organizational structures. (http://education.stateuniversity.com/pages/1859/Colleges-Universities-Organizational-Structure.html)

The Board of Regents or Trustees is often made up of political appointees or other highly influential people who then have the responsibility of governing the university or system. The board does not typically control or interfere with the daily operations of the university. Rather, it is involved with the impact of legislation and external forces on public higher education. The political influence can have significant positive or negative effects on how education is delivered and on the work life of faculty and administrators. Board members may not have any experience with higher education, personally or professionally, and this lack of expertise can negatively influence their decision making.

A public university is led by a chancellor or president who answers to a system president or chancellor. The chancellor of the university is responsible for the overall and day-to-day function of the university and is the ultimate decision maker for the university. He or she works with the provost, the chief business or financial officer, and other vice chancellors or vice presidents to conduct the business of the university. The chancellor is the face of the university and is frequently engaged in fund-raising and appealing to the Board of Regents or Trustees and to legislators on behalf of the university. Before you accept a leadership position, try to determine how the chancellor/president and provost interact with other leaders in the university. If possible, determine whether they "have the back" of the deans. This is vitally important and if it is not the case, then you may find yourself trying to follow through on directives only to find that your superiors change course every time faculty raise any objection.

The chancellor or president is likely to have a cabinet chosen by him or her to help with decision making. They may choose to include whomever they believe can bring the most expertise to the discussions. However, the vice chancellors/vice presidents are usually included. Depending on the chancellor or president, they may also choose to meet regularly with deans, shared governance groups, and other representatives.

The provost or vice president of academic affairs is in charge of academic affairs. Consequently, the SON and the chief nurse executive report to the provost. The provost typically works with associate and assistant provosts on issues pertaining to academic affairs. Although the faculty and faculty senate are responsible for the curriculum, the provost is responsible to the chancellor for the quality of the education delivered and the efficiency and quality of the academic colleges/schools. Consequently, the registrar and the library often answer to the provost as do the deans, academic advisors, and others who have direct impact on academics and student success. However, some roles might fall under a vice president or vice chancellor for student affairs as would anything pertaining to student life, such as residence halls, the student health center, student clubs, and possibly the dining facility.

FACULTY AND FACULTY SENATE

Faculty govern the curriculum. Typically, in public institutions, faculty are represented by the faculty senate or council. The senate has bylaws and may follow a very prescriptive procedure to run meetings. Deans in SON are usually full-time administrators who may teach. They are not faculty. However, chairs or directors of programs or program tracks may be part-time administrators and thereby retain their faculty voting rights. Deans frequently sit as ex officio members of faculty committees, even within the SON. They do not get to vote in these committees or in the senate.

Faculty are the core of a public university and can wield considerable influence on university and SON decisions. The wise nursing administrator will strive to work closely with faculty and request their input whenever possible. Sometimes the administrator has to make decisions for the good of the SON without faculty input, but these occasions are rare and the administrator should try to be transparent about why faculty could not be involved.

Public institutions and SON vary with regard to the committee structure. Typically, curricular issues are reviewed and approved within the SON but then must obtain approval from a faculty senate curriculum committee. Similarly, certain policies, such as SON bylaws, may have to have faculty senate approval. Faculty senates vary as to how much control they maintain over what individual schools or colleges do within the university.

One common function of the faculty is to review other faculty for promotion and tenure and sometimes reappointment. The SON faculty review faculty within the SON who are due for promotion or tenure and make a recommendation to the dean. The dean's recommendation is then submitted to the provost, who makes a recommendation to the university chancellor or president. Eventually, the Board of Regents or Trustees reviews the recommendations for tenure and promotion and makes the final decision. Reappointment decisions, such as those for adjunct instructors or for faculty still on the tenure track, often end with the provost.

Faculty rank typically proceeds from assistant professor to associate professor to full professor. SON often have a "clinical track," instructors who may hold a practice doctorate or a master's degree who are a level above clinical instructors or adjunct instructors. Those on the clinical track may or may not have requirements for service and scholarship and, if they do, the scholarship requirement is often considerably less than that it is for faculty. Clinical-track instructors typically have rank and receive a higher salary than clinical instructors and adjuncts, but less than faculty. Clinical instructors, by contrast, are frequently adjuncts, people who are hired on a semester or annual basis to fill gaps in the curriculum. They may teach anywhere from one course to a full load of courses and usually do not have service or scholarship requirements. Clinical instructors typically do not have rank but are vital to the SON because of the clinical expertise they bring to the classroom and student clinical experiences.

The tenure track is typically 5 to 6 years in length with the expectation of applying for tenure in the sixth year. This means that all work toward tenure must be completed within 5 years. Experienced faculty or those previously tenured can often negotiate years toward tenure. For example, an experienced faculty hired in a new university might negotiate and receive up to 3 years toward tenure because his or her record of teaching, service, and scholarship is lengthy and strong. This means that he or she would have 2 years at the new university to demonstrate continued excellence in teaching, scholarship, and service before applying for tenure. Only faculty with a good chance of receiving tenure should negotiate for "years toward tenure" because if refused tenure, faculty typically have 1 year to find another job before leaving the university. The individual may have the opportunity to switch to the clinical track, but this is not guaranteed.

Requirements for reappointment, promotion, and tenure vary depending on the mission of the university and SON so explore this before taking a position. Also, faculty workload, such as number of credits one is required to teach, expectations for service and scholarship, is key because these expectations will give you an idea of how to prioritize your time to achieve goals toward promotion and tenure.

The concept of shared governance will be threaded throughout this book within discussions about the public university perspective. Shared governance is a key concept in public universities and applies to the amount of input and involvement faculty, adjuncts, students, and even secretarial or support staff have in university decisions. There are likely to be senates or councils for part-time or adjunct faculty and for support staff.

These shared governance groups will have representatives on many SON and university committees.

Shared governance, in theory, is a wonderful idea. It allows varied perspectives from stakeholders and helps administrators make informed decisions that can benefit everyone. It can also be overplayed. Faculty, in particular, may feel that they should have a say in every decision but this is neither wise nor practical. Administrators make decisions every day and cannot always wait for input from faculty who often disagree with each other. In addition, faculty are experts on the curriculum but frequently know little about budgeting, assigning courses, system policies, or other nuances for which administrators are responsible. It is difficult for faculty to make informed recommendations on everything when they do not have the background or "big picture."

Students typically have a university student organization and a student-nurses' association (SNA). The types and level of activity depend on the particular institution. However, SNA typically engage in activities that support the SON and the community. The leaders of the SNA can be important allies for SON administrators by assisting with communication to students and ensuring that student concerns are addressed.

UNIVERSITY OFFICES

Institutions vary but public universities are typically organized to include a variety of departments. Academic affairs, led by the provost or vice president/vice chancellor of the university, encompasses faculty, the schools or colleges, the registrar, the library, and other departments directly related to education. There may be a department of student affairs that oversees student-related services such as residence halls, admissions, campus police, the student health center, and athletics. The chief finance or business officer is likely to oversee an administrative office that develops and/or approves contracts and budgets. This office may also be responsible for risk management, security, and facilities management. There may also be a division related to fund-raising or development and directed by a vice president (see Chapter 4). Public universities organize different departments within these divisions or units based on their mission and strategic plan but you should know which departments fall into which unit or division and who is ultimately responsible for each division. It behooves new administrators to seek out and meet these people shortly after starting the job and to maintain these relationships.

There may be tension or friction between the administration and faculty because administrators are tasked with making the decisions that will impact faculty and faculty may perceive that they have less influence on those decisions than they should or could have. A strong chancellor/

president and provost can help unite both factions to work together and bring their strengths to the table. They must also know when to include shared governance and when it may not be appropriate for the good of the university.

SON STRUCTURE

The structure of the SON within a public institution can also vary considerably. Nursing may be a department within a school of health professions or health sciences. It may be part of an academic health center that includes a medical school and possibly other professional schools such as pharmacy and physical therapy. If nursing is a department, it is likely to be led by a chair who reports to a dean of the school. If nursing is its own school or college, then it will be led by a dean. Within schools or departments of nursing, there is typically further breakdown into undergraduate and graduate programs and even further into emphases or tracks. For example, in the undergraduate program, there might be a traditional BSN track and an accelerated track (students with previous degrees who seek BSNs). SON may choose to include RN-to-BSN programs under the undergraduate or graduate umbrella. Associate degree nursing programs, while all undergraduate, may also break themselves down into departments depending on their size. A graduate program might have a family nurse practitioner track and an administrator track but students in both tracks receive a doctor of nursing practice (DNP) degree. There might be tracks within the masters in nursing program, as well.

The undergraduate and graduate programs are typically led by a director or chair (a director is usually subordinate to a chair) who reports to the dean or chair of the department. The director or chair of the undergraduate or graduate program may have an assistant director or vice-chair. Some universities break it down further and have coordinators for each of the levels in the nursing program, such as junior-level and senior-level coordinators. Each of the programs might have a clerical assistant or secretary who supports the program and work–study students who also assist.

There is typically at least one associate dean who may assist the dean to oversee the entire SON or who may have special designation, such as the associate dean for research or the associate dean for academic affairs. Assistant deans may work with the associate deans either in special areas or to support each program. SON may have centers such as the center for research or the center for community engagement. SON tend to develop centers around what they want to be known for as doing better than anyone else and for which they have faculty expertise.

SON and nursing departments require a lot of support staff who may or may not be academics. In addition to faculty and instructors, a school or department may have a lab coordinator, a simulation coordinator, clinical placement coordinator, and study abroad coordinator. There may be an in-house budget analyst and a human resources coordinator. Keep in mind that budget considerations—which increasingly impact public universities and colleges—may change the structure described here. There may be more overlap of roles in an attempt to conserve resources.

Clerical or secretarial staff are invaluable. They often have history with the university and can be especially helpful to new faculty and administrators regarding formal and informal chains of command and communication. They often know how to get things done. Support staff can make or break an SON. The ability of staff to work together as a team, cover for one another during sick time or vacations, and work for the advancement of the school mission can make all the difference in accomplishing the work of the SON. Infighting and competition can stifle their creativity and delay progress significantly. Support staff should be encouraged to feel as much a part of the SON as the faculty as the SON cannot thrive without them. They should be encouraged to think of innovative ways of enhancing efficiency and success. Administrators and faculty should show their appreciation often and generously (Figures 1.1 and 1.2).

Work–study students can be very helpful and may or may not be nursing students. They can run errands and make copies, perform Internet searches, and type reports. Check institutional policies regarding whether they can have access to student-related information.

■ THE FOR-PROFIT UNIVERSITY PERSPECTIVE

For-profit colleges and universities use a variety of organizational structures depending on the size of the student body, the number of campuses, the number of states where campuses are located, and the requirements of the accrediting agency. However, the majority, if not all, follow a business model as opposed to an academic model. The purpose of any business is to make money for the owners and shareholders by selling a product. In the case of for-profit schools, the product for sale is education. This business model is often perceived as valuing operations over academics, as there is a strong focus on admissions and retention and the employees who work in those departments. It is logical that schools that rely entirely on tuition for income would focus on having robust admission and retention numbers, yet proprietary schools are often criticized for this, the implication being that if you care about money you cannot care about quality. The criticism is not logical nor is it justified in most cases (Deming, Goldin, & Katz, 2012). Furthermore, all colleges and universities, whether they are public, private,

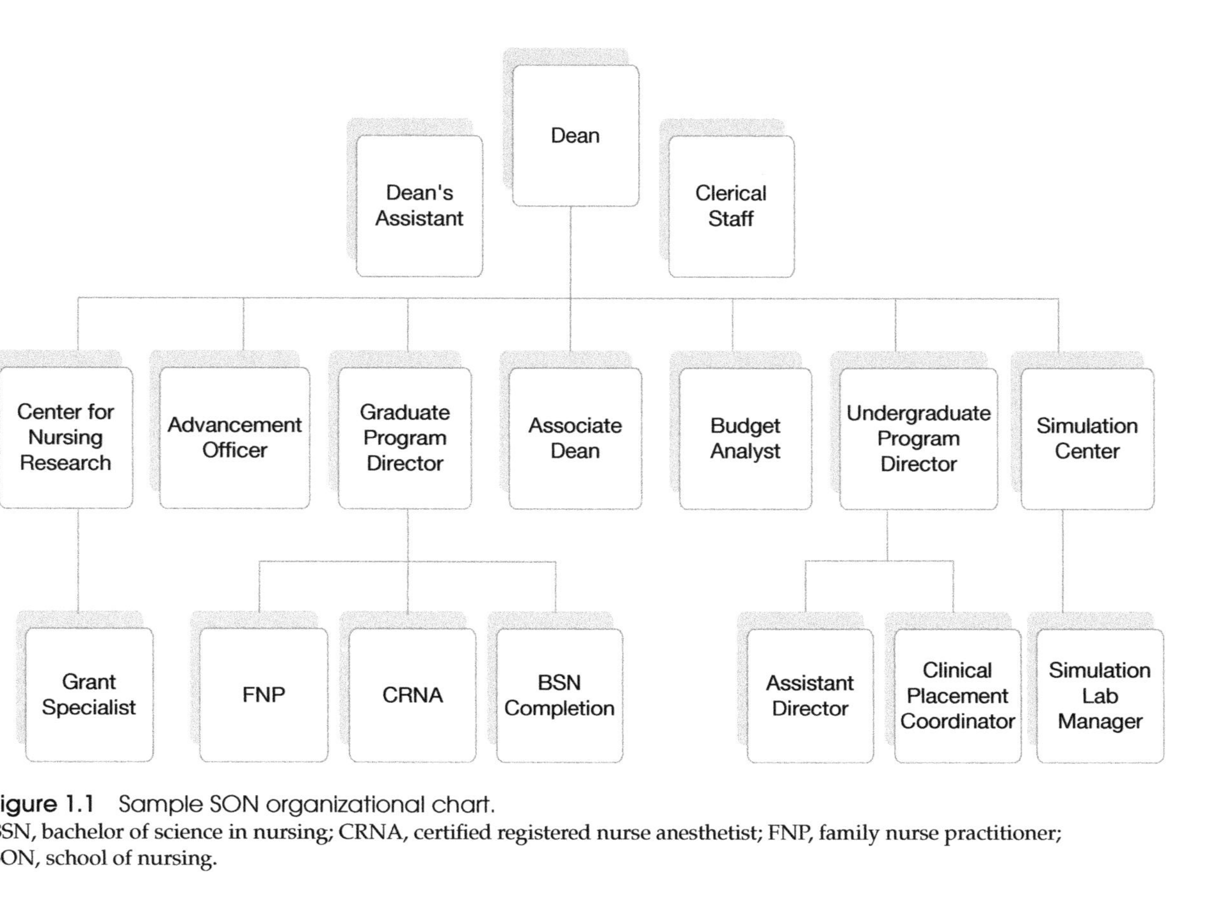

Figure 1.1 Sample SON organizational chart.
BSN, bachelor of science in nursing; CRNA, certified registered nurse anesthetist; FNP, family nurse practitioner; SON, school of nursing.

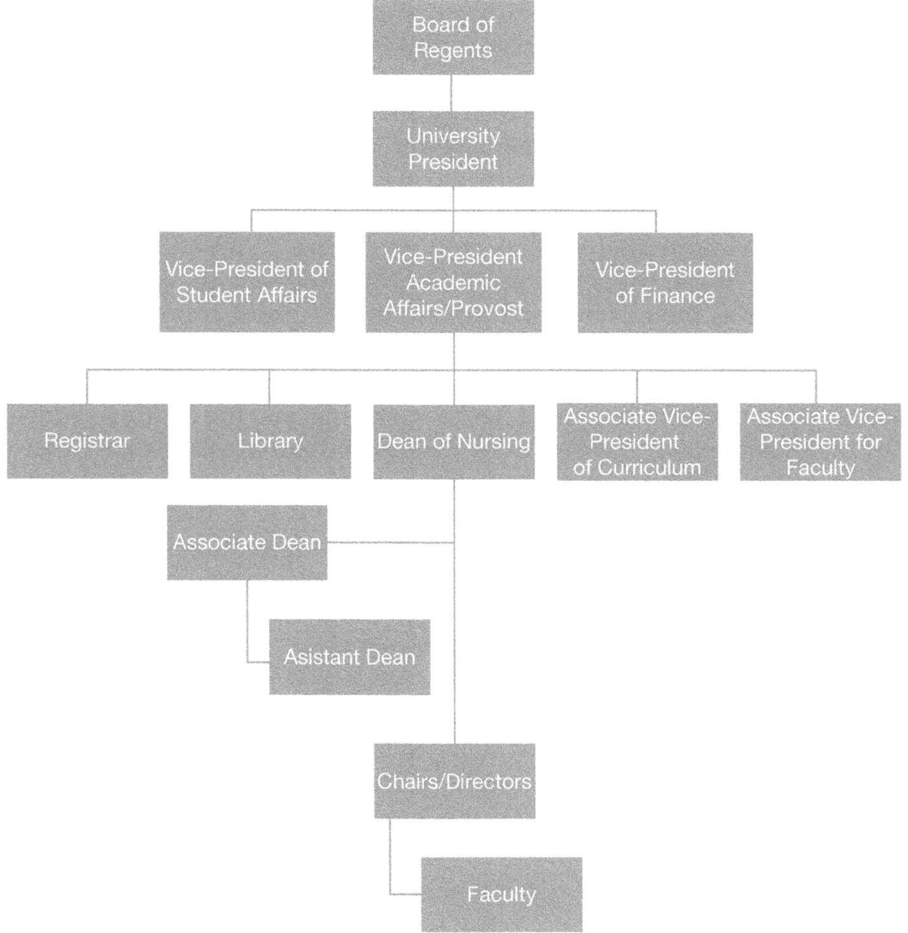

Figure 1.2 Sample public university organizational chart.

or for-profit, not only apply fiscal and personal resources to recruitment and retention but are also held accountable for outcomes in both areas. There are operational reasons for paying attention to admissions and retention but a major reason is that both regional and national accrediting bodies have standards related to retention and graduation rates for all schools.

Public and private colleges and universities enjoy revenue streams other than tuition, such as research grants and endowments, which are often tied to academic quality so these organizations do not focus as much on admissions, but a dip in enrollment is a concern across all educational institutions. The type of accreditation the college has obtained drives outcomes. As discussed elsewhere, many proprietary programs are accredited nationally and national accrediting agencies focus heavily on retention and placement. As a result, the chief operating officer (COO) is often the highest ranking administrator with traditionally academic departments, such as the registrar and student services, reporting to that office. Some for-profits have both a COO and chief academic officer (CAO) who report to a university president. Others have the CAO reporting to the COO, and some may not have a CAO at all. In this case, determine how academic decisions are made and by whom. On the other hand, many proprietary schools, especially the large national schools, have regional accreditation that requires both a CAO and a board of supervisors. These programs are just as focused on student academic achievement as their public and private not-for-profit counterparts and dedicate significant resources to support student success.

Organizational structure also determines reporting relationships, the formal opportunities for shared decision making, and the agility in which the organization can respond to new ideas and initiatives. This is where proprietary schools have clear advantages over their nonprofit counterparts. Most for-profits operate lean organizations with flatter structures and are typically able to respond to data and information more quickly than the bureaucracies common to public and private institutions. Figures 1.3 and 1.4 illustrate some of the more common organizational structures used in for-profit organizations. The most inclusive, albeit most challenging, design is the matrix structure. In a matrix organization, thought leaders are organized around product lines at the national or state level with input from thought leaders on the campuses who coordinate via technology to collaborate and make decisions. Although not as cumbersome as bureaucracies, the matrix organization is not as agile

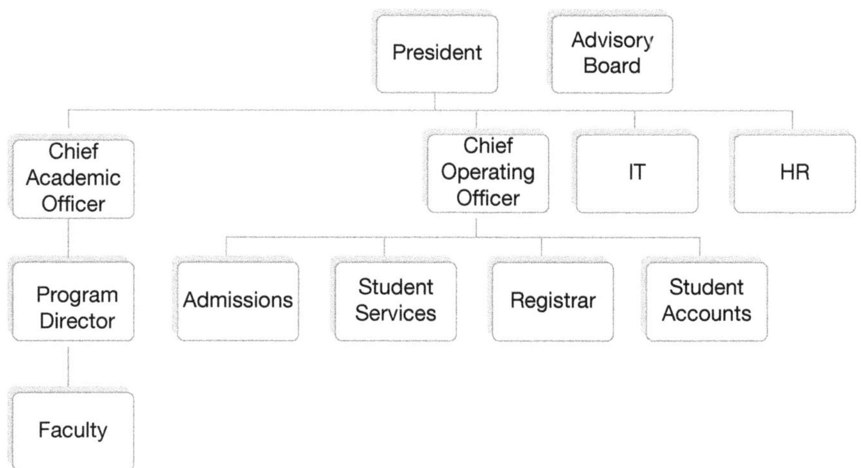

Figure 1.3 Simple stand-alone organizational structure of for-profit school of nursing.
HR, human resources; IT, information technology.

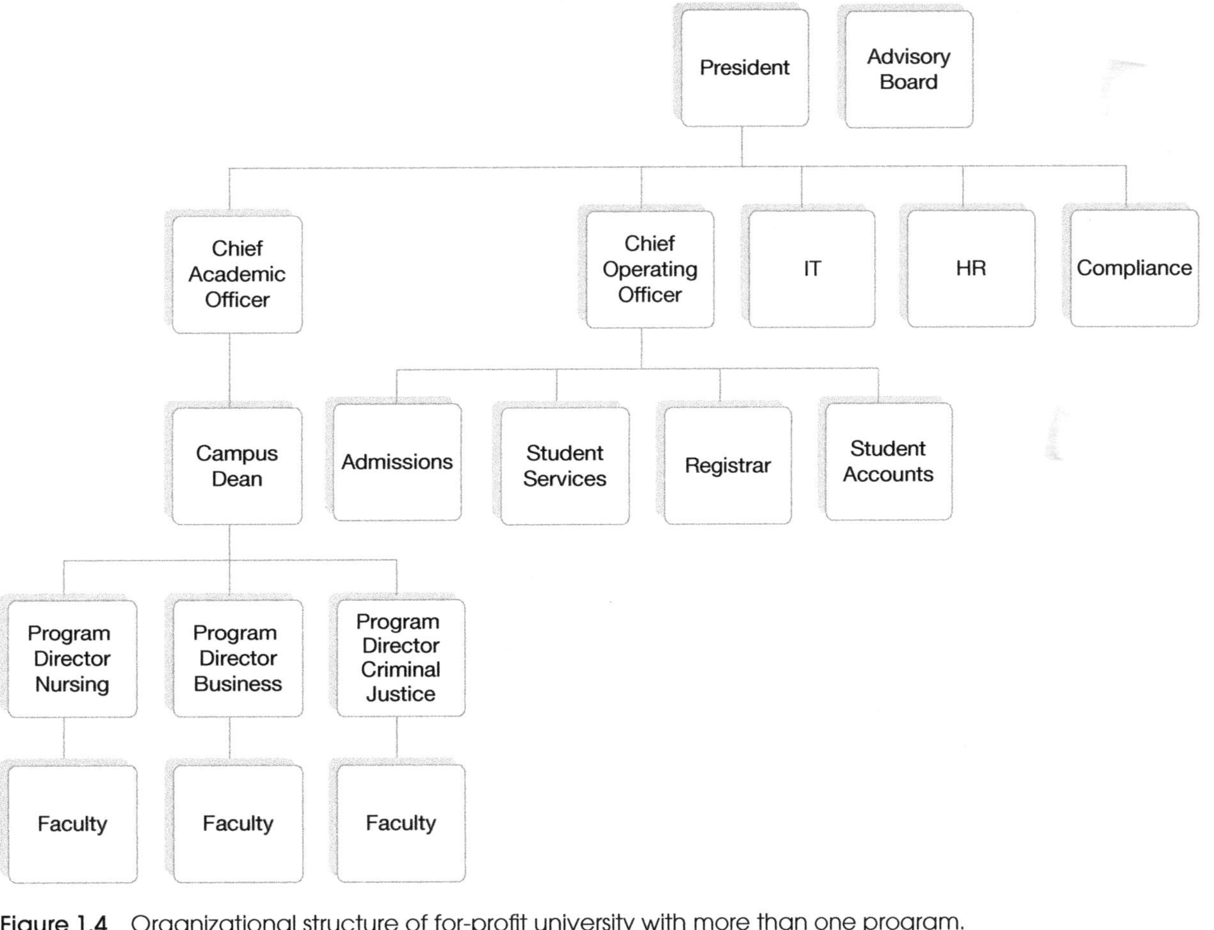

Figure 1.4 Organizational structure of for-profit university with more than one program. HR, human resources; IT, information technology.

as the flatter structures and you do have to guard against "siloing" the product lines.

Decision-making structures vary based on the number of programs offered, the number of campuses, and the number of states where programs are offered. As you might imagine, navigating the requirements of different state boards of nursing requires a very strong compliance team. Large national organizations typically utilize compliance teams to assist with decisions that affect program structure, curriculum, and faculty, whereas small, one-program schools may leave all decision making to the dean or director. Schools with a number of campuses in a single state may use academic councils to align policies and ensure consistency across campuses.

FACULTY/FACULTY GOVERNANCE

Each school or college will operate somewhat differently, but in most cases there is no faculty council or senate that is empowered by a set of bylaws to vote on university-level decisions in the same manner as public and private entities. Schools that use a centralized national curriculum tend to have a national-level person who oversees academics and a team that works on curriculum. In many organizations, faculty are not involved in the development stage, but do have opportunity for feedback. Faculty generally have control over their own practice and course assignments, but may have little control over the syllabus or how the course content is presented. Reporting structures within the SON depend on the number of faculty. Small programs (80 students or less) will likely have a program director or dean and two or three full-time faculty members. Larger programs will have an assistant dean or director and 10 or more full-time faculty. Remembering that the number of full-time faculty in the proprietary sector is small (as few as four) and the percentage of adjuncts is fairly high (60%), there are usually very few faculty members available to participate on committees or serve as course coordinators. Therefore, reporting structures tend to be less formal in smaller programs.

Faculty hiring and advancement is usually managed with limited input from faculty themselves. Smaller programs may have the dean or director interview faculty and put a team of other directors together to watch a teaching demonstration. Larger programs typically involve the faculty in the hiring process, but whether or not they get a chance to interview candidates depends on the philosophy of the dean/director. Most, if not all, proprietary programs are nontenure-track programs and many do not use contracts for employment. If there are different levels of compensation, represented by different titles, these are earned by meeting criteria related to scholarship, teaching excellence, and service to the organization. Faculty may participate in the promotion process in some schools and may have no voice in others. The for-profit sector varies more in policies related to promotion and decision making in general and you should ask specific questions at any school for which you are considering employment.

Some nursing programs face challenges with acquiring the faculty needed. This is especially true in a school that offers many disciplines as you are competing for budget and resources with programs that typically rely even more heavily on adjunct faculty and may only have one or two full-time faculty, who also have administrative responsibilities. Fortunately, state boards of nursing have regulations related to nursing faculty that can be used as leverage if needed. One benefit of colleges that provide only nursing programs is that the CAO is a nurse who understands what is needed to provide a quality education. Always ask what the credentials of the CAO are and what his or her experience with nursing programs has been (see, e.g., Figures 1.3 and 1.4; Table 1.1).

Table 1.1 Example of Simple Matrix Structure Used by Multisite Single-Program Colleges of Nursing

National President				
Regional Director	**VP of Admissions**	**VP of Academics**	**VP of Marketing**	**VP of Student Services**
Campus A president	Campus A admission director	Campus A dean	Region 1 director of marketing	Campus A director of student services
Campus B president	Campus B admission director	Campus B dean	Region 1 director of marketing	Campus B director of student services
Campus C president	Campus C admission director	Campus C dean	Region 2 director of marketing	Campus C director of student services
Campus D president	Campus D admission director	Campus D dean	Region 2 director of marketing	Campus D director of student services

VP, vice-president.

UNIVERSITY OFFICES

Again, there is some variation in the offices found in proprietary programs. The typical offices include admissions, student accounts, student services, career services, and registrar. Student services and career services are often combined. There usually is no student health or stand-alone office to assist students covered by the Americans with Disabilities Act (ADA). Student accounts and financial aid are usually combined. Some larger schools might have a compliance office and/or an office of institutional effectiveness. Most do not have a research department but may have an institutional review board (IRB) within the office of institutional effectiveness.

SON STRUCTURE

The variety found in the organizational structures of public universities can also be found in the for-profit sector. One determining factor is whether or not the college or university offers programs other than nursing. When the SON is located in a large university that offers programs other than nursing, the structure of the SON will reflect the larger organizational structure. For example, if the university uses the term "director" for heads of programs, the head of the SON will be called a director. Most for-profits do not use titles like "chair" and there are usually two few faculty to oversee to warrant more than one administrator. When the college decides to open a school the first faculty member hired is generally considered the "program lead" and this title remains until there are sufficient courses and faculty to warrant a promotion to director. The SON may be required to use a different titling structure if the board of nursing in that state requires specific terminology.

While all employees must meet human resource requirements, the job descriptions for nursing faculty will be expanded, again, based on the state board requirements. For example, many state boards require that a nursing faculty committee determine who gets accepted to the SON and this will appear in the job description. Some state boards require that there be a separate dean or director for each campus offering nursing courses, regardless of the distance between locations. For-profits are reluctant to do this as it creates added expense not found in other programs. As an SON director you must know the state regulations and be strong in enforcing them.

SON that are stand-alone programs typically have large student bodies and therefore larger numbers of faculty and staff. These programs tend to break down functions similar to large public universities and use titles, such as provost, dean, associate dean, and so on. They are also likely to have directors for other areas, such as labs, tutoring centers, and student services, all of whom report to the campus president who is generally a doctorally prepared nurse.

The number of faculty required at clinical, classroom, and administrator levels contributes to the factors that make nursing very expensive to operate. To be more cost-effective, smaller organizations will look to save money by sharing support personnel. It is common for these organizations to have one administrative assistant who serves all of academics.

Faculty and program leaders keep their own calendars and produce their own materials, including instructional materials and exams. Large programs typically have a department that handles regulatory matters, including compiling documents, which may fall to the faculty in smaller programs. If the faculty is made up of three or four persons, then the work usually will fall to the director with minimal support. Similarly, committee work, even recording minutes, will have to be done by faculty. Ask these questions early. I am reminded of the newly hired program director who asked where her administrative assistant would be located only to find out that she did not have one.

All of the federal rules that apply to the public and private sector also apply to the for-profit schools. Therefore, they are also eligible to use federal work–study students. Again, how these students are used varies from institution to institution. You can see that there are a number of reasons to discuss the organizational structure and decision-making structure as it relates to mission and implementation of that mission.

■ PRIVATE UNIVERSITY PERSPECTIVE

Organizational structures at private universities may differ depending on the size of the university, the foundational tenets of the university, and whether or not the university is faith based. For example, faith-based organizations will have governance relative to the faith or church that will play a significant role in setting policy and even having a say in academic programming. For example, this author's university is affiliated with the Lutheran Church Missouri Synod (LCMS) and is also a part of and under the supervision of the Concordia University System (CUS). The CUS includes 10 colleges and universities across the United States. The presidents and senior leaders at each of the 10 colleges are all active LCMS members. Theology faculty at each school have more specific requirements and are approved by the CUS Board of Directors before being appointed or called to the school. Each school within the system is overseen by a Board of Regents and it is mandatory that Board of Regent members are active members in good standing of LCMS congregations.

Board of Regent members are elected by the Synod. The university president is the executive leader of the Board of Regents.

In a private university affiliated with the Catholic faith, a Board of Trustees and officers representing the Catholic Church may select a president using a search committee made up of key stakeholders. The president typically must demonstrate a lifelong commitment to Catholic education and must show commitment to the university's core values that align with the Catholic faith. In some cases, priests or nuns may be appointed as Catholic university presidents. Priests and nuns may serve as part-time or full-time faculty. It is not uncommon for private universities affiliated with the Lutheran faith to have ordained ministers in a variety of positions in addition to president and faculty, including serving as deans, registrars, or directors of advancement.

The Board of Regents or Trustees at a private university typically has ultimate authority and responsibility to determine all university policies. However, the Board of Regents or Trustees will often delegate administrative matters to the president and the president's administrative council, and academic matters to a senior vice-president of academics or a provost. Like public universities, private universities will have administrative councils in which administrative leaders, headed by the president, include various vice-presidents, and assistant vice-presidents, such as those leading strategy, finance, information technology, student success, student life, marketing, and athletics, among others. At this author's university, the president is appointed for a 5-year renewable term and is the leader of the administrative council. Typically, the faculty chairperson and the student government leader will be included in the administrative council. In faith-based organizations, a campus pastor or priest may be part of the administrative council. The administrative council coordinates and oversees matters related to administration of the university; that is, the business side of the university. The administrative council will often give input on academic programming, particularly as it relates to potential budget implications, impact on current material and human resources, and association with student life.

Handbooks at private universities may include administrative policies, which are those that do not need faculty input for adoption, revision, or repeal. As noted, a faculty chairperson or faculty senate chairperson often sits on the administrative council to provide faculty input and perspectives. The same is true for a student government representative who sits on the administrative council and who can provide the students' perspective on pertinent matters. However, administrative council decisions are often made based upon not only the financial well-being of the university, but also are made taking into full consideration the mission of the university. For example, an academic program that might be market driven and could be financially sound will not receive administrative council approval if it is at all contrary to the university's mission. Effective administrators are transparent, using open communication regarding administrative decisions, particularly those that directly affect faculty and staff. Although faculty may believe they should have input into these decisions, the bottom line is that faculty often do not have all the details relevant to the overall function of the university and elements necessary for its ongoing success. Faculty should take a great interest in such information when it is available to them, as they should similarly and equally take an avid interest in the overall success of the university.

Like public universities, private universities will have academic councils, comprised of various vice-presidents, assistant vice-presidents, and deans who coordinate and oversee matters related to academics and the curriculum within schools and programs at the university. Academic councils may include leaders who oversee distance or online learning. If there are off-campus centers where the university offers classes and programs, leaders of these centers may also be a part of the academic council. The academic council will debate and recommend academic and curricular matters to the faculty through whatever structures are in place for such approvals. For example, new academic programs, program revisions, and course changes are typically initiated by a particular school or schools, and then they may be reviewed and approved by a curriculum committee, faculty senate, or the entire faculty, as well as by the academic council.

Both the administrative council and the academic council provide oversight as related to overall accreditation, as well as accreditation of individual programs that are overseen by deans and department chairpersons or directors. Accreditation standards take into account both the academic rigor of courses and programs, as well as the means by which the programs are available to and delivered to students. Academic programs must have the appropriate content as well as the appropriate resources to be successful. Therefore, both of these bodies work collaboratively to ensure that accreditation standards are attained and maintained.

Faculty have responsibility for the curriculum (teaching) and matters related to research and scholarship. Faculty are expected to collaborate with administrative leaders and staff to facilitate cocurricular activities and ensure they are compatible with the university's mission. At this author's organization, the faculty authority currently lies with the plenary faculty, that is, all faculty who hold a full-time appointment within the university. This structure worked well for many years until the university experienced exponential growth in the student body, which also resulted in comparative growth in faculty numbers. This growth was never paralleled by updates to the faculty governance structure. Currently, with more than 300 full-time faculty members, conducting business and getting programs and courses approved with all 300+ members weighing in and voting can be daunting. Therefore, efforts are currently underway to strategically revise the academic governance structure.

The current faculty senate at this author's university has limited authority and responsibility, and does not represent each school equally. Deans, who also hold faculty status at the university, can be members of the senate. In fact, deans currently make up a disproportionate number in the faculty senate membership compared to the faculty members. The current faculty senate chairperson, who serves as chairperson of the plenary faculty, is working to revise the administrative structure to give the faculty senate more responsibility and authority to deliberate, vet, and approve proposals related to curricular matters. The goal is to revise the university's bylaws; so there is equal representation on the senate from each school. This smaller representative body could have much freer discussion and debate on curricular proposals and other matters related to the curriculum than when trying to discuss issues in an auditorium with more than 300 faculty members present.

Because it is so closely tied with the curriculum, faculty may also have control over assessment related to curricular matters. There may be SON and university assessment committees that ensure the curriculum meets program and student learning outcomes. Sometimes, depending on the size of the university, there could be separate graduate and undergraduate assessment committees both at the SON and university level.

Private schools will tout their traditions of academic excellence tied to a strong sense of mission. It will be commonly noted throughout this book that at private universities, mission is at the core of every curricular, cocurricular, and administrative policy and decision. Therefore, each individual faculty member has the responsibility of carrying the mission forward. Promotion in rank and achieving tenure (in those private universities that have a tenure system) ensures the university of a faculty member willing to commit to this mission. Deans and department chairpersons will work diligently with new faculty members to provide mentorship regarding expectations for promotion in rank and achieving tenure. Faculty handbooks should clearly outline the expectations and requirements for promotion and tenure. At some private schools, only full-time faculty may be granted tenure, and those serving in administrative roles may not be eligible for tenure status.

At some universities, all faculty within the SON may be asked for input on recommendations to the dean regarding a peer's qualifications for promotion or tenure. At other schools, only faculty who have achieved advanced rank or the rank for which a faculty member is striving to achieve are involved in giving recommendations on a faculty member's advancement or tenure status. In some private schools, there may not be recommendations made at the SON at all, but rather the first level of recommendations may be made by a university committee made up of representatives from all schools. Whatever the mechanism for approval (or nonapproval) at the SON level, recommendations for promotion and tenure will then typically move up the chain of command to the dean, then to a university rank-and-tenure committee, then to the vice-president of academic affairs (or provost), next to the president, with final approval by the Board of Regents or Trustees. Working through this system, promotion, and tenure decisions will often take a full academic year before a final decision is announced. Universities will have appeals processes in place for faculty who are not awarded the promotion or tenure they were seeking.

Just like in public universities, when private universities have a tenure system in place, faculty have a set number of years in which to achieve the milestones for teaching, scholarship, and service (e.g., 7 years). If faculty do not meet the qualifications, typically a 1-year terminal contract will be awarded after which time the faculty member is dismissed. If a school has a nontenure clinical track in addition to a tenure track, it may not be possible to switch tracks once hired into one or the other. For example, if a faculty member was hired to a tenure-track position and then did not meet the qualifications for tenure, that faculty member may not be allowed to switch to a nontenure track for the reasons of not meeting the tenure qualifications. Rather, she or he may be given a 1-year terminal contract and would be dismissed after the terminal contract is fulfilled. One reason for this inability to switch tracks is that SON may have a certain number of allocated tenure and nontenure track positions. Just because a faculty member does not meet the expectations for the tenure track, it does not mean there would be an open position for which she or he could be inserted onto the other track. The fact that the faculty member did not meet expectations for one track may be a good reason to move the faculty member along so that he or she can find a position that better suits his or her professional goals.

Sometimes faculty have misconceptions that the merit of their teaching or years of service may be enough to be granted tenure. Unless all three areas of teaching, scholarship, and service are met, tenure will not be granted. Similarly, at private schools, tenure could be withheld if the faculty member demonstrates behaviors that are not consistent with the school's mission.

Administrative positions within the SON and the university are often granted for a limited term. For example, administrative terms might be for 1-year renewable, based on the supervisor's recommendation. For faculty with administrative responsibilities, the administrative aspect of the contract may be for 1 year, whereas their corresponding faculty appointment can be variable, depending on whether or not there is a tenure system in place or another structure for renewable contracts. For example, assistant professors may have 2-year contracts, associate professors may have 3-year contracts, and professors may have 5-year contracts.

Various committees will be in place to carry out the work of the university. Bylaws or policies will denote committee purpose, responsibilities, and membership composition. Often the goal is to have each school or college represented on each committee. Large schools like arts and sciences may be awarded more seats (members) than smaller schools within the university for some committees, similar to the U.S. House of Representatives. This type of structure can lead to voting blocks that could cause the smaller schools to lack a clear and distinct voice. This is why a senate system, with equal representation from each school, is more highly favored.

Typically, deans, along with directors or chairpersons, have both administrative and academic oversight in their schools and departments. For example, deans, directors, and chairpersons work collaboratively recruiting faculty and staff and recommending their hire, evaluating their performance, and recommending continued employment. They also work collaboratively overseeing curricular and academic matters related to their programs. All will typically be expected to work within a set budget, and adding any new faculty or staff positions would need administrative approval. Capital expenditures over a certain dollar amount may have to go through a university approval process. Budgeting and resource allocation are addressed in more detail in Chapter 8. Curricular and academic decisions are initiated within the school, but as mentioned previously, may need approval all the way up to the Board of Regents or Trustees. SON administrators ensure programs within their school meet accreditation standards.

In addition to administrative and academic councils and SON and university committees, SON often have advisory councils that do not have "voting power" but may have significant input into school decisions. Advisory council members are often selected by the dean and should include representatives from healthcare organizations and systems that employ graduates of the school's programs. Other key stakeholders should be included who may have a finger on the pulse of healthcare and who can give input into current and future needs of curricula and programs. Members may have a key stake in the university's mission and they will provide input into operationalizing the mission. Student representation on the advisory councils is important.

Organizational charts vary. Harvard is one of the most well-known private schools in the United States and its organization chart (https:// oir.harvard.edu/fact-book/org_chart_central) has the administrative sector on one side and the academic sector on the other side, with key individuals in the middle who report directly to the president. The Board of Overseers and Harvard Corporation are included but not connected to either sector.

Marquette University's organizational chart is rather unique in that is has a circular design with three key members in the middle of the circle: the president, provost and executive vice-president of academic affairs, and executive vice-president of operations. Direct reports for each of the academic affairs and administrative side of the university make up the outer boundary of the circle (see www.marquette.edu/leadership/documents/ULC-org-chart.pdf). One cannot help but note that the circular depiction of Marquette's organizational chart distinctly illustrates the concept of mission at the core of everything.

Organizational structures in private universities vary considerably related to the size of the organization and its student body, the numbers of academic programs, and even perhaps according to the methods by which programs are delivered (there may be separate structures for online vs. face-to-face programming). Learning about the organizational structure of an SON and a university may seem "boring" when seeking an administrative or faculty position. It may take work to look for this information on the website. When interviewing for a position, it is wise to ask about how administrative and academic decisions are made and the ease in which such decisions are made. Have a sound understanding of the organization structure, as this structure will dictate how business is conducted and work in the SON is completed. Without this understanding, an academic leader may walk into a position not knowing how to carry out the role responsibilities for which he or she has been hired. Moreover, it is possible that an academic leader or faculty member could take a position in which the organizational structure and how work is done is directly contrary to personal desires or beliefs in how best to accomplish the role responsibilities.

REFERENCES

Deming, D., Goldin, C., & Katz, L. F. (2012). The for-profit postsecondary school sector: Nimble critters or agile predators? *Journal of Economic Perspectives, 26*(1), 139–164.

Organizational Chart-Central Administration. (n.d.). Retrieved from https://oir.harvard.edu/fact-book/org_chart_central

CHAPTER 2

APPLYING FOR/SEEKING A NURSING FACULTY POSITION

It may be helpful to readers to read both this chapter and Chapter 3 to learn more about seeking a position in academe. Although Chapter 3 focuses more on the pursuit of a position in academic nursing leadership, much of the content will be helpful to readers seeking a faculty position. Conversely, aspiring academic leaders will find content in this chapter helpful as a foundation for the content in Chapter 3. The reader should note that this chapter is structured differently from the others because much of the information overlaps all three types of universities and because there are many common considerations when seeking a faculty position.

Think carefully about what you are looking for in a faculty position. There is a shortage of nursing faculty, particularly doctorally prepared nursing faculty, so you are in the fortunate position of having a wide variety of choices. Therefore, approach this endeavor using a deliberative process.

■ THE PUBLIC UNIVERSITY PERSPECTIVE

Although most schools of nursing (SON) are anxious to hire faculty, public university systems invariably suffer from reduced funding.

Hiring costs money. Expenses include advertising, travel reimbursement for candidates, meals, lodging, and start-up costs such as office equipment and technology (Perlmutter, 2016b). According to Perlmutter, "the optimum hire becomes somebody who will say 'yes,' who may not cost as much, who will remain for more than a few years before leaving for (perceived) greener pastures. In short, a good fit" (p. A22). He lists a few questions that professors should ask themselves before applying for a position and that hiring authorities are likely to ask themselves about the candidate:

- Are you going to be too expensive?
- Are you going to be a flight risk?
- Will you succeed with our students?
- Will you fit into our faculty culture?
- Where did your degree come from?

If you are just considering pursuing a doctoral degree with the goal of becoming faculty, then choose your program of study and graduate school very carefully. Degrees from for-profit doctoral programs are often considered less rigorous than those from nonprofit programs. As you consider the options, do your homework thoroughly. For example, keep in mind that although public systems of higher education share many similarities, they differ with regard to policies and procedures that may be unique to the system. Faculty tend not to concern themselves with these policies until they start working in a university within the system and encounter a particular issue that requires them to study the policies. Public systems tend to have many policies and processes that can cover almost any imaginable situation. Many policies are developed and maintained by the faculty and others are mandated by a Board of Regents or senior administrators from throughout the system who work together to standardize policies. It is unrealistic to expect that prospective faculty can acquaint themselves with most or all of these policies. However, faculty seeking a position in a public university should attempt to learn about certain policies and procedures that are likely to pertain specifically to the faculty role. One can either locate these regulations on the system website or ask the SON how to find them. Review the system, university, and SON policies. They may differ but university and SON policies cannot be inconsistent with system policies.

Read about the mission, vision, and values of the university and the SON. Do they resonate with you and your perspective and goals? If the strategic plans are available online, read them, too. Is there an orientation and ongoing mentoring?

■ THE FOR-PROFIT UNIVERSITY PERSPECTIVE

All of the factors listed in the public sector discussion should be taken into account when contemplating a position in a for-profit institution. However, you should understand the "worldview" of the organization as it underpins the mission and frames all decision making, including hiring. Many for-profit organizations started out as career schools or colleges offering diplomas and certificates, which then evolved into degree-granting institutions. Ask whether the institution considers itself a career college and by whom it is accredited.

Many career-focused institutions have moved to regional accreditation but some still have national accreditation. National accrediting organizations focus primarily on outcomes related to retention and employment and may view learning outcomes as indirect measures of effectiveness. Most for-profit institutions (and some community college programs) must meet federal regulations related to gainful employment, which only heightens the emphasis on being employed rather than getting a quality education. The two are not mutually exclusive, and many for-profit schools provide programs that match or exceed the quality of public programs. The point is that you should be aware of the history, framework, and philosophy that underpin the mission and vision of the sector in general and the organization in particular. This is especially true if you are moving from the public sector or a school with regional accreditation as it truly is a different playing field.

As a result of their history, these organizations may still have a career preparation focus rather than an academic focus. This leads to a desire to hire "experts" in the field with current practice experience. Teaching experience is a plus, but not necessary. This has positive and negative aspects. On the positive side, this opens the door for nurses who have discovered through their practice that they love to teach but cannot find classroom positions in traditional universities. On the negative side, nurses with no experience in classroom management are often thrust into the classroom totally unprepared. The career mind-set and interest in hiring those with current expertise lead to the practice of hiring adjuncts instead of full-time faculty. Full-time faculty are expensive and often are not highly valued. In fact, employees working on the operations side of the organization may have better compensation packages than do the faculty. Ask about salaries and the ratio of full time to adjunct positions not just to determine whether the school meets your needs but to gain insight into its view of academics. If you are uncertain about the organization, consider beginning as an adjunct and moving into a full-time position. If you are looking for a full-time position, information related to the for-profit sector is provided in the following sections.

■ THE PRIVATE UNIVERSITY PERSPECTIVE

When investigating a faculty position at a private school, there are many considerations, but thoroughly investigating the mission and foundational tenets of the organization is critical. All faculty must be considered a good "mission fit" with the organization. Faith-based institutions are allowed to hire based on religious preference, and the hiring process may require an interview with the president or a member of the Board of Regents to ensure mission fit. Some faith-based organizations may require a certain percentage of faculty are of the like faith. At the organization in which this author works, all faculty members must be Christian and active members of a church. This is nonnegotiable, even for adjunct faculty who are hired to teach one course only. Faith-based schools may require that potential faculty and staff are members of the affiliated faith and may even have a quota for the number of faculty who must be practicing members of a church. Private schools that are not faith based may require potential faculty and staff to demonstrate in some way a connection with the mission or affiliation with the foundational beliefs. There may be additional policies related to behavioral expectations consistent with the mission, even outside of work, for which a faculty member must agree to adhere.

COMPARING PERSPECTIVES

What follows is a list of topics with which the prospective faculty candidate should acquaint him- or herself. Compare and contrast these between and among the universities and SON you are considering pursuing.

SHARED GOVERNANCE

Shared governance refers to the degree to which faculty have a say in what happens within the system or university. Does the university have a faculty senate or council and do representatives to the senate or council represent the university at system meetings? How much say do faculty have within the university? Ask others how productive the faculty senate or council is? Do they tend to lag in getting anything done or do they listen to their constituents and move things along?

■ THE PUBLIC UNIVERSITY PERSPECTIVE

Although its scope of shared governance varies, even within public university systems, shared governance is one of the hallmarks of employment at a public university. The focus of shared governance may be primarily on faculty, but in some systems secretarial staff and adjunct faculty may also have representation. Ask faculty whether they feel they have a strong voice in university and SON decision making. Try to speak to adjuncts and secretarial or support staff to see whether they feel represented. Interpreting their responses really depends on how important shared governance is to you and whether you would like to have a voice in SON and university politics. Even if it is not significant to you, you will want to be sure that your interests are well represented by the faculty who do participate in shared governance opportunities. Be aware that as either faculty or an administrator, shared governance can hamper decision making and convolute decision-making processes. If all but very minor decisions must go through several layers of approvals, then the likelihood of accomplishing something in a timely way can be decreased substantially.

■ THE FOR-PROFIT UNIVERSITY PERSPECTIVE

There are many variations of shared governance throughout the sector. Institutions that have a corporate structure with many campuses, especially those that have campuses in more than one state or U.S. territory, tend to have centralized processes and curricula. This structure makes true shared governance challenging. However, there are always opportunities for faculty to have a "voice." Faculty typically voice their concerns, ideas, needs, and so forth at regularly scheduled faculty meetings. Faculty also have a voice in all decisions related to admissions and progression of students. There are as many different formats for faculty input as there are programs. Large or multisite programs generally provide templates or report forms for faculty to respond to or complete. Even when processes are centrally developed and disseminated, faculty at the local level may determine how those processes are rolled out locally. Be certain to explore how local decision making takes place as well as how communication and collaboration are effected with national or regional decision makers.

■ THE PRIVATE UNIVERSITY PERSPECTIVE

Degrees of shared governance are common in private organizations, similar to public universities, and faculty typically have a strong voice in academic matters. The level of their input into administrative matters varies, as some private universities can be more hierarchical when it comes to administrative decisions. However, this can allow private universities to more quickly change programming to be more responsive to stakeholder needs and the changing academic climate. Faculty typically have a significant say in the curriculum, as they are the content experts. Problems can arise when faculty become embedded in the "way we always did it" and less aware of emerging trends in their fields, and that can hamper curricular evolution. This may be more common in private organizations that do not have a strong emphasis on scholarship and research for their faculty and less common in organizations that have a stronger emphasis on these areas. Sometimes asking questions about the liberal arts core and how its effectiveness is measured or when the nursing curriculum was last updated or revised can give you a sense of change and how readily it is accomplished.

The level of say that faculty have in matters may not be evident when reviewing printed materials. If the faculty handbook is available online, reviewing committee structures and their makeup may shed light on the amount and level of involvement faculty have in shared governance. See what committees on which faculty are represented, review the committee election or appointment process, and what the functions and responsibilities the committees have to get a sense of faculty voice. Sometimes private schools can have very vocal and "regulating" alumni groups and/or bodies related to the school's founding organization or sponsors. Check to see how involved the Board of Regents or other administrative councils may be in day-to-day operational matters or in curricular decisions. There could be some restrictions that align with the school's mission or foundational doctrines of which potential employees of that school should be aware.

PROMOTION AND TENURE

■ THE PUBLIC UNIVERSITY PERSPECTIVE

What are the university and system policies for tenure and promotion?

Typically, the system sets the policy but universities and SON within the system are allowed to develop their own policies as long as they are not inconsistent with the system policies. Consider these questions: How long does it take to become tenured? What is the process and timeline for promotion and tenure reviews? Does one have to be reappointed every year? Does reappointment occur every 2 years as one moves through the tenure track? What are the expectations to obtain tenure, such as producing a certain number of peer-reviewed publications, presentations, awarded grants, committee work, and involvement in professional organizations and on executive boards? Is there a policy regarding posttenure review?

Is there a mechanism, such as a faculty development grant, to support faculty to conduct research or complete a project? How well developed and staffed is the Office of Sponsored Programs? This is the office that helps faculty apply for and manage grants.

Faculty often feel somewhat beholden to the senior faculty who may be involved in recommending them for tenure or promotion. Junior faculty may worry that they must not disagree or upset senior faculty who could influence their careers. If possible, get a sense from current or former faculty whether the promotion and tenure process has been perceived as fair and equitable.

Are there guidelines and resources one can use while on the tenure track? For example, will you be assigned or be able to choose a tenured faculty mentor? Are there seminars or tutorials available on campus or will there be financial support for you to attend national conferences to help you become a better researcher or scholar?

Support for conference attendance is key because it is hard to learn about being a faculty or to be able to present research findings if conference attendance has little or no financial support. What is the process for applying for support or is each faculty allotted a certain amount of money per year for conferences?

The system is likely to have an umbrella policy for travel reimbursement, such as a cost per mile and other guidelines. The SON will need to pay travel reimbursement out of its budget and travel costs related to clinical site visits and conferences can be considerable. Know how much leeway the administrator has regarding travel reimbursement. Also check on whether your move, should you be offered and accept the position, will be reimbursed in part or in full. Defer this question until you are offered the position. However, the website might have information about standard reimbursement for moving expenses (Box 2.1).

Box 2.1 Public University Promotion and Tenure Considerations

- What is the process and timeline for tenure reviews?
- What are the expectations and guidelines for tenure?
- Are there faculty development grants or other university grant support?
- What level of support can you expect from the Office of Sponsored Programs or the campus grants support office?
- Does the SON have personnel or financial resources to support faculty research and projects?
- Is the promotion and tenure process considered fair and equitable?
- Is there a faculty mentor to guide you?
- Is there financial support for conference attendance? How much? What is the process?
- What is the travel reimbursement policy?

SON, school of nursing.

■ THE FOR-PROFIT UNIVERSITY PERSPECTIVE

Although tenure is not common in the for-profit sector, there may or may not be a process for moving up in rank. In many instances, there are only two faculty positions available: full time or adjunct. In schools in which this is the case, promotion does not occur in rank, but in position. For example, there is no move from one level of instruction to another, but from faculty to program leader. This promotion is usually made on the basis of the number of students or programs in the school. A few large programs do have a process for promotion in rank. This process mirrors that found in public and not-for-profit institutions. Faculty desiring a promotion in rank must submit a portfolio that demonstrates they have met the designated criteria. These institutions may also require faculty to attain a certain rank, such as "master instructor," before being considered for leadership positions. One size does not fit all in this sector so explore this area carefully.

■ THE PRIVATE UNIVERSITY PERSPECTIVE

A tenure system may or may not be in place at private schools; that is something to ask about and consider. If there is a tenure system, applicants should review the criteria to achieve tenure and what the expectations are for teaching, scholarship, and service. At smaller private schools, a greater focus may be on teaching; scholarship expectations may be less than one might see at a public university. However, when seeking a faculty position, applicants want to inquire about how current faculty stay up to date in their fields of study and how that is assessed. There can be specific service expectations at private schools that align with the school's mission. At a faith-based Christian school, service to the church may be expected. At other private schools, service to the affiliating organization may be expected.

Whether or not a tenure system is in place, applicants should ask how promotion is handled. Is there a faculty committee or an administrative committee that reviews those seeking promotion or is the decision made by the dean or other senior administrator? If there is a committee that handles promotions, the committee is often made up of those members who hold advanced academic ranks. Like public universities, senior faculty members may have a significant say in the promotion of junior faculty. Promotion may be tied to years of service at the organization. If an applicant has worked at another school, he or she may want to ask about credit for years of service coming from that other job to achieve a promotion sooner than if the years of service must be at the school in which the applicant accepts a position.

REAPPOINTMENT

■ THE PUBLIC UNIVERSITY PERSPECTIVE

You may be interested in applying for a faculty position that consists only of teaching or teaching and committee work, commonly known as *service*. Perhaps you are applying for a non-tenure-track position. If so, what are the requirements for reappointment? Is the workload heavily skewed to teaching clinical classes or is it a mix of clinical and theory classes? What are the expectations for scholarship, service, teaching, and travel?

Very important to the faculty role and your interactions with others within the SON and the university is whether there is collective bargaining and, if so, the terms of the contract. How, when, and by whom you will be evaluated are critical. Also, if not reappointed or awarded tenure, do you have a year after receiving this news to conduct a new job search?

■ THE FOR-PROFIT UNIVERSITY PERSPECTIVE

Faculty in for-profit schools do not, as a rule, sign contracts or receive specific appointments. Faculty agree to teach on a term-by-term basis based on the need of the program and the credentials of the faculty member. These agreements may be formalized in written agreements or statements of assignments but either party can decide not to honor the agreement. For example, if a course is under enrolled, it will not be offered and the agreement with the faculty member is null and void. This can be frustrating for the faculty member. Similarly, the faculty member may decide at the last hour that he or she is unable to keep the agreement. This creates a great deal of distress for the school who will be challenged to find a qualified replacement. Faculty not teaching in any given term are considered inactive. Faculty who make it known that they are leaving the organization are evaluated in terms of eligibility for rehire at the time of termination.

■ THE PRIVATE UNIVERSITY PERSPECTIVE

For private schools, especially those that do not have a tenure system, applicants should ask about reappointment and how that process works. Some may have contracts of varying lengths for those of differing academic ranks. For example, an initial appointment may be 2 years for all new faculty hires. Academic rank is determined by the applicant's qualifications and prior accomplishments based upon the school's criteria for each rank. There may be a rolling-contract system in place. For example, assistant professors may have 2-year contracts, associate professors may have 3-year contracts, and professors could have 5-year contracts. A rolling contract means that each year that the faculty member remains in good standing based on the annual performance evaluation, a "year" is automatically reloaded onto the contract. So, the person always has a 2-, 3-, or 5-year contract in place as long as she or he is good standing. If faculty are not performing up to expectations for the role, a performance-improvement plan can be initiated. Reloading that year of the contract may be withheld as one motivating criteria for the faculty to improve his or her performance. Once conditions of the improvement plan are met, that year can be restored.

When faculty members are granted promotion, the new contract length would be awarded. Administrative positions may be for 1 year only, or a shorter length of time than the faculty contract. For example, a dean with the rank of professor could have a 5-year faculty contract, but the contract for the dean role would be for 1 year and not automatically renewed.

Although rolling contracts such as described here do not provide the long-term security that holding tenure may provide, they do afford faculty members some guaranteed time within the organization, which offers significant stability and job security. Of course, contracts can always be broken for cause, that is, if the faculty member is deemed to have behaviors or actions that were in violation of policies, procedures, or expectations of the faculty role. Similarly, if faculty pursue another position, they are not held to the length of the contract. Thus, the rolling contract does provide stability, but it also allows faculty to pursue other opportunities if desired, without consequences. Contracts and length of terms for reappointment can be as varied as private organizations are. Applicants are encouraged to ask questions to get a good understanding of the terms of initial appointment and specific criteria necessary for reappointment.

Remember that most faculty have, at one time, worked as nurses in the private sector. Although those who came from healthcare organizations in which unions were in place had contracts and seniority protections as part of their employment, most nurses work without any sort of contract. Census days off and other layoff days were common based on patient census and other scheduling conditions affecting healthcare organizations. In the business sector, people do not have the benefit of a contract in most jobs and performance is evaluated continually as part of ongoing employment. Therefore, although you should thoroughly understand the conditions of employment, many nurses who come into academe are surprised if they get only a 1- or 2-year contract upon initial employment. Yet, the reality is that many have worked for years without any sort of contract in place and were truly "at-will" employees, unless they were part of a union. Bottom line, performance excellence will likely keep you employed, no matter what the setting, unless significant budget cuts affect staffing levels.

WHAT IS THE UNIVERSITY LIKE?

Take time to review the university website and delve beyond the attractive face pages that are designed to draw students, parents, and prospective faculty to the university. Look at whatever the university has allowed the public to see.

■ THE PUBLIC UNIVERSITY PERSPECTIVE

Are there a lot of activities going on at the campus? Are there visiting professors and international trips for students and faculty? Are there mechanisms throughout the university for continued faculty learning? Are university orientation sessions offered to new faculty? Is there specialized training for teaching online? Perhaps lively and successful sports teams are important to you. Take a look at that, too. What athletic teams are supported and do athletic teams get more of the money and resources than do the academic colleges? What other activities exist for students?

Are there photos of students and faculty from diverse backgrounds? All universities should strive for diversity so the university is enriched by a variety of perspectives. Are there lesbian, gay, bisexual, transgender, and queer (LGBTQ) student groups and opportunities for worship by people from a variety of belief systems?

Check whether there are human interest stories about what faculty, staff, and students are doing. Is there a strong emphasis on community engagement? Does the university have a theater or concert hall open to the public? Think of what matters to you in your work life and specifically explore the opportunities available to you on campus.

If possible, locate the university's strategic plan. Review the mission, vision, and values of the university. Do you think your goals and interests will be a good fit?

■ THE FOR-PROFIT UNIVERSITY PERSPECTIVE

For-profit colleges and universities tend to be housed in a single building. The program itself may be located on a single floor. This does not mean that there are no activities for students and faculty, but it does mean that space for activities is limited. Ask about ceremonies such as pinning, graduation, sport events, and mixers? Where are those located? Are you expected to attend?

Look at the mission and vision of the institution, are they aligned with your values? Some mission statements are student centric, others are focused on career development. Ask about the mission and whether there is a values statement.

Ask specifically about orientation. Most for-profit programs operate on an 8- to 10-week term with no breaks between terms. Therefore, if you are hired just before the start of a new quarter, there is likely to be little or no orientation to the role or the program. Seasoned faculty who have "been there, done that" cope fairly well in this setting. However, if you are new to the role, you will likely become overwhelmed. Schedule your start date so that you have time to be oriented and, if possible, observe or team teach with other faculty. It is particularly useful to shadow a clinical instructor if you are new to the clinical faculty role. Simply receiving an agency orientation to the clinical site and unit is not sufficient. Ask about mentoring, master instructors, and other resources available to you.

■ THE PRIVATE UNIVERSITY PERSPECTIVE

What has been written about public and for-profit universities is also applicable to private institutions. When reviewing the university website, look for activities that align with the mission and foundational tenets of the organization, which is likely a reason affecting your decision to explore job opportunities there. Do you see a good match? Most private universities take pride in "living their mission" and making it evident to students, prospective students, community members, and other internal and external stakeholders. For example, are there mission trips or other service opportunities for faculty? As you look at the pictures, can you see the mission in action? Private schools may have specific orientation programs that allow faculty and staff to delve deeply into the university's history and mission and expectations for living the mission in all encounters both inside and outside of work. This would be in addition to a typical mandatory orientation for faculty, which introduces them to abundant resources for teaching and for professional development, to faculty governance and committee work, to scholarship expectations and resources to support scholarly endeavors, and to relevant policies and procedures. The orientation also typically introduces new faculty to campus leaders. As part of their initial contract and contract renewal, faculty at some private universities are required to sign an agreement, detailing expectations for carrying out the school's mission.

Prospective faculty members should ask about reimbursement for professional development and what types of activities might be covered.

Many private colleges often have some sort of tuition reimbursement, remission, or allowance for faculty and their family members. For example, if a private college is looking to increase the number of faculty with terminal degrees, there may be tuition assistance available. Sometimes, faculty members' children or spouses can get reduced tuition at the university in which the faculty member is employed or at schools within their system. Because salaries at private colleges are often lower than comparable salaries in the public sector, tuition reduction for children or spouses can amount to a significant dollar amount that can make up for a slightly lower salary. Some faculty specifically seek out positions at private universities so that their children can attend these schools for reduced or free tuition.

Find out the contract period; are faculty awarded 9-, 10-, or 12-month contracts or some variation of that? Are all faculty awarded the same length of contract or are there options to have a 9-, 10-, or 12-month contract? If there are options, what are the ramifications for pay periods? For example, if faculty are awarded 9-month contracts, can they be paid over 12 months, or do they just get paid over 9 months? For nurses used to being paid every 2 weeks, it can be a real shock to get paid once a month.

What are expectations for being physically on campus or working from home? Are these policies written or "unwritten"? At the university in which this author works, there was a written policy that all faculty have 10 face-to-face office hours per week. As online courses and programs became more commonplace and some faculty were actually teaching 100% online courses, that policy had little meaning for those teaching online. Even faculty who taught face-to-face classes were finding that the typical 8 a.m. to 5 p.m. time to add office hours was not always convenient for students, especially those in the SON who have several clinical days away from the university. Faculty were finding a much greater connection with students when they had virtual office hours using technology associated with the school's online learning management system in the evenings or even on weekends. The policy was amended to be less restrictive as to the face-to-face requirement and noted that faculty had to have 10 hours dedicated to scheduled office hours per week. The format for the office hours was left up to faculty based upon their teaching load and their students' needs.

Another example of policy change at this author's school was related to using vacation time. Faculty are awarded 20 days of vacation per year as part of their 12-month contract (this is in addition to having "off" during spring break, a university 2-day fall break, and days over Thanksgiving and Christmas when the university is closed). A policy was in place that vacation could only be taken during the summer months. Although the intent of this policy was such that faculty could not take vacation when they had teaching expectations, the reality was that there were several programs in which classes were offered during times that were different from the traditional academic calendar. These classes and programs had courses in the summer and some that ran over spring or fall break. Taking vacation only in summer did not meet these faculty members' needs. Therefore, the wording of the policy was amended such that it stated that vacation time could be used during times in which the faculty member did not have teaching responsibilities.

WHAT IS THE SON LIKE?

It may be beneficial to take some time to review the SON web pages.

■ THE PUBLIC UNIVERSITY PERSPECTIVE

Review the SON mission, vision, and values. They should be consistent with the university mission, vision, and values. Does the SON utilize a conceptual framework? It is worthwhile to review the SON strategic plan and student and faculty handbooks, if these are available. It is worth asking whether you can be permitted to see them. These and the accreditation self-study report can give you a very good idea of the history and current status of the SON. However, they may not be shared with outsiders. If you cannot access these documents, see Box 2.2 for some questions to ask (in no particular order).

The NCLEX® (nursing board exam) pass rate and graduate certification pass rates should be visible on the web pages. These pass rates offer a good indication of how well the SON is doing educating its students. Be sure that the SON is not on probation. You can also look at the state board of nursing website to check the status of the SON.

Student handbooks are interesting and worthwhile reading. There is usually a handbook for each program level (undergraduate and graduate). How detailed are these policies and when were they last updated? When you are interviewed for the position, try to learn how closely these policies are followed or whether significant exceptions are made. For example, most SON have strict written policies about whether a student can fail a class and remain in the program and the characteristics of the appeal process. However, in actuality, faculty may be especially sympathetic to students who fail a course and make exceptions to the rule instead of the other way around. Often unbeknownst to faculty, this can open the school to lawsuits (if exceptions are made without extenuating circumstances).

A review of student handbooks for a technical standards policy is also helpful. The Americans with Disabilities Act Amendment (2008) requires that schools accept students on their merit and qualifications and provide reasonable accommodations if and when a student requests them.

Box 2.2   Public University: Considerations to Explore Within the SON

- What is the policy on intellectual property for faculty?
- What about courses you develop while you are employed?
- Do you own them or does the university?
- With which clinical sites does the SON partner?
- What is the employment rate for new graduates and alumni?
- What is the staff-to-student ratio in theory and clinical classes?
- Do faculty teach clinical classes or are adjunct faculty hired to teach clinical classes?
- What is the credit load for faculty and what justification must be provided to obtain credit releases?
- What support is provided by the SON for research and scholarship?
- What is the admission policy for nursing students?
- What is a passing grade for nursing students?
- What is the student appeal process?
- What is the student grievance process?
- Can students fail more than one course in the nursing program?

SON, school of nursing.

Therefore, to refuse admission solely due to a disability is illegal. While on the subject of disability, be aware of the legal term *sovereign immunity*. This means that, in states that have not waived sovereign immunity, an employee of a public organization *cannot* sue the state. Consequently, a disability claim brought against a public organization is likely to lose.

Take a careful look at the SON website. Unfortunately, sometimes even the best SON do not necessarily keep their web pages up to date. However, accredited SON are required to ensure accuracy and consistency of the web pages and other public documents. Many schools wait until accreditation is due to update these materials. If the initial SON web pages are difficult to navigate, that may or may not be a clue to the success of the SON. It may require you to dig deeper to glean the information you need about the SON.

■ THE FOR-PROFIT UNIVERSITY PERSPECTIVE

The information provided for public institutions is applicable to the for-profit sector. In some cases, nursing is the only program offered so there is no variance between the university policies and those of the nursing program. In others, there are a variety of both health-related and non-health-related programs offered across the spectrum of degrees that may be granted. Nursing programs tend to be more rigorous and have narrower, stricter policies for admission and progression. It is a good idea to discern where the commonalities and variances lie and the extent to which those differences are valued and adhered to. Some for-profits have very little infrastructure and may rely on standard operating procedures rather than formal policies and policies may be developed ad hoc or after some incident occurs. Due to their agility, institutions in the sector tend to change policies as they grow and expand. Ask whether there is a policy manual and/or committee that oversees them. If the school is part of a multicampus system, do policies have to be the same across campuses? You might think that consistency across campuses is a given but it is not, especially when campuses are in different states and under different board of nursing regulations.

■ THE PRIVATE UNIVERSITY PERSPECTIVE

In addition to learning about the university and SON policies as noted earlier, at private schools, look for unique things that may be related to "culture" that may be influenced by the foundational tenets (Box 2.3).

Learn not only the policies that govern student and faculty behavior, but also personnel policies that may affect vacation time, leave, and insurance coverage.

Potential applicants should also ask about how clinical teaching works within the faculty load. For example, typically within SON, there can be a 1:3 or 1:4 ratio for clinical credit-to-clock hours (one credit of clinical equals 3 or 4 hours of clinical time). When seeking a faculty position, questions should be asked about how faculty are awarded teaching

Box 2.3 How SON Culture May Be Connected to Mission

- Are service activities expected related to a specific cause or mission?
- Are there opportunities for mission work locally, regionally, nationally, or internationally?
- If a faculty member supervises a mission trip with students, can that work be considered part of the faculty load or is that part of service to the school or university?
- Are there religious holidays that are celebrated for which classes would not be in session? For example, at a faith-based school, classes or clinicals may not be in session on Good Friday and Easter Monday.
- Does the school close over Christmas break?

SON, school of nursing.

credits for clinical. For example, if faculty teaches a three-credit clinical, are they awarded three credits in their teaching load or are they awarded contact hours (nine credits). At some schools, there could be other variations, such as six credits awarded when teaching a three-credit clinical. Applicants should ask about those policies as they will affect scheduling and workload. Similar questions should be raised if potential faculty could be teaching in the skills or simulation lab and how teaching credits are awarded for that aspect of a teaching load.

Potential applicants should inquire about class sizes, particularly in the SON. Private schools often tout that having smaller class sizes makes them unique and more student centered as compared to public organizations. They may advertise "guaranteed" graduation in 4 years because classes are accessible to complete majors during that time frame. However, in the SON, when clinical groups are typically capped at eight or 10 students, sometimes didactic courses are expected to have larger numbers, to help balance the budget. Therefore, the smaller and more intimate didactic classes may not be the reality in the nursing major.

Potential applicants should ask about expectations for teaching across programs (traditional undergraduate, bachelor of science in nursing [BSN] completion, accelerated, and graduate) and across delivery methods (face-to-face, hybrid, or online). If an applicant is not accustomed to teaching online, for instance, one should ask about the professional development opportunities to familiarize oneself with best practices in this area. If an applicant is especially interested or has qualifications better suited to one program (undergraduate or graduate) or one delivery method, this should be expressed.

One aspect associated with teaching loads that may be more difficult to ascertain is how oversight for doctor of nursing practice (DNP) projects or PhD dissertations are assigned. Is this an expectation for all doctorally prepared faculty? Is this considered a part of a teaching load, or is it considered service? Is there remuneration for this responsibility? How many students might a faculty member be expected to oversee during a typical academic year? Overseeing these projects can take a considerable amount of time, and there should be some sort of allowance within the teaching load or some aspect of payment associated with such responsibilities.

WHO IS THE CHIEF ADMINISTRATOR?

■ THE PUBLIC UNIVERSITY PERSPECTIVE

Look at the SON website to see whether there is information about the chief nurse executive (CNE). Is this person a nurse or is nursing housed within a department in a college or school led by a chief administrator from another discipline? The chief nursing administrator might be a director or chair or could be a dean of the SON. Look at the credentials of the CNE. If her or his curriculum vitae (CV) is available, look for how long the CNE has been a nurse and in nursing education. Has the CNE been faculty? If so, she or he may have a greater understanding of the faculty perspective. If he or she has been a CNE for a long time, he or she may be quite removed from the faculty role. In larger public institutions, deans especially often have so many staff members, including associate and assistant deans, chairs, and directors, that their contact with issues important to faculty may be minimal. If you cannot find information about the CNE, that is not a good sign. However, you should be able to find basic or additional information by googling the person's name.

■ THE FOR-PROFIT UNIVERSITY PERSPECTIVE

The board of nursing in most states will require that the program is overseen by a nurse. However, if the program is one of many programs within a health sciences or health professions department or college, the dean or director of the department/college may not be a nurse. If this is the case, proceed with caution. Equally important, but harder to determine, is the type of experience the dean/director has in both education and nursing practice. For-profits tend to hire DNPs and doctors of education (EdDs) as opposed to PhDs. The degree granted reflects the pathway to higher learning. Either may be appropriate for the current needs of the school, but they are not the same and you need to determine whether your philosophy aligns with that of the leadership. Talk with faculty about the school's responsiveness to nursing needs, where leadership's focus is, how nursing salaries compare to those of other programs, and how clinical time is compensated and accounted for in workload calculations.

■ THE PRIVATE UNIVERSITY PERSPECTIVE

Aspects already noted for public and for-profit universities apply to private organizations as well. At smaller private universities, there may not be a separate SON, but nursing may fall under health sciences or another school. See whether the leader of the SON is a dean or a department chairperson. The chief academic officer's title could indicate his or her level of influence within the school.

WHO ARE THE CURRENT SON FACULTY AND STAFF?

Look at the SON website for information about the current SON faculty. Some of the questions in the sections that follow might not be answered by reviewing the web pages and may need to be asked during phone or on campus interviews.

■ THE PUBLIC UNIVERSITY PERSPECTIVE

What is the faculty turnover rate? What do faculty think of the leadership within the SON? This author once taught at a university in which 10 faculty voluntarily left their positions in the first 2 years of their employment. It was clear that faculty were not happy with the leadership. Later, the author became aware that this was common knowledge about this particular SON but the author had not known or bothered to ask the questions. Because one of the roles of the search and screen committee (SSC) is to try to convince you of what a great place the school is to work, committee members are unlikely to give you straightforward answers to these questions. However, the astute listener and observer can pick up on cues that all is not necessarily rosy or, conversely, that people are genuinely happy working in the SON. If you know of or can locate someone who previously worked at the school, ask this person to give you honest feedback about the culture within the SON. If people are reluctant to talk, despite your assurances of confidentiality, then that should be a clue that there may be problems.

What level of education do SON faculty have? Do their CVs indicate involvement in scholarship and publication? What about service to the SON, university, and profession? Do you see yourself fitting in with these faculty? Are there more adjunct or part-time instructors than full-time faculty or tenured and tenure-track faculty? If so, ask why. In public education especially, budget restrictions may force administrators to hire more part-time instructors than full-time faculty because the university does not need to pay benefits for very part-time (below 0.5 full-time equivalent) instructors. Also, SON must have instructors who have current clinical expertise; if full-time faculty are not current, the gap may need to be filled by part-time instructors who also work clinically.

Box 2.4   Public University: SON Faculty and Staff

- What is the faculty turnover rate?
- What level of education do the faculty have?
- Do faculty engage in current research/scholarship?
- Do faculty have current publications in peer-reviewed journals?
- How many support staff exist within the SON?
- What kind of support do staff provide to faculty?

SON, school of nursing.

How many support staff are included in the SON? Look at the titles of the support staff. This may provide clues regarding whether faculty must perform the bulk of their own clerical work or can rely on staff support. Try to locate the SON organizational chart to see how flat or hierarchical the organization is and who works directly with or for whom (Box 2.4; see Chapter 1 for a discussion of organizational structure).

■ THE FOR-PROFIT UNIVERSITY PERSPECTIVE

It is unlikely that faculty will be listed on the university website so you will have to ask about them directly. The number of full-time faculty is very small in the for-profit sector, in some cases as few as three. Adjuncts are used to teach both theory and clinical courses and some of these may have been part of the team longer than the full-time faculty. Ask about all faculty members' strengths and weaknesses and how they get along. How much experience do they have? Typically, they will have a lot of practical experience but very minimal teaching experience and almost no experience with curriculum development. Credentials are determined by the state board of nursing but be careful to examine the type of master's or doctoral degree earned.

A major difference in the makeup of the faculty is that the majority will be prepared with master of science in nursing degrees and a high proportion will be new to teaching. Ask about how long the current faculty has been there and the mix in terms of content expertise. The number of full-time faculty tends to be small so you must determine your fit. In very small programs, there may be a single section of the course you are teaching, which means support may be limited. Administrative support is likely to be minimal and probably shared. There are certainly benefits to working with a small close-knit group such as agile decision making and more rapid implementation. But the downside is there are fewer people to actually do the implementing.

In terms of staff, the SON will, in all likelihood, share staff with other colleges or departments.

■ THE PRIVATE UNIVERSITY PERSPECTIVE

Faculty at private organizations must value the university's mission. That is one aspect that ties faculty to each other and may make them less diverse than you might find in a public university. Do full-time faculty have terminal degrees? If not, is there an expectation for achieving a terminal degree within a certain period? If a majority of faculty do not have terminal degrees, it is likely that research and scholarship may not be a high priority. From what institutions do the faculty hold terminal degrees? Do they hold terminal degrees from research-intensive universities or from for-profit or other organizations? Again, this can be an indicator of the level of scholarship that will be produced. You have to determine what your career trajectory is and whether that matches with faculty who are already employed there.

For those considering a move to academe, and considering advanced education as part of that move, you should consider *where* you will enroll to earn your advanced education. It may be wise to consult with leaders at SON where you may desire employment for advice prior to choosing a program. For example, most state boards of nursing require that faculty hold a minimum of a master's degree in nursing to teach nursing. Within baccalaureate and higher degree SON, a doctoral degree is often preferred or required. Therefore, some nurses who have chosen to get a master's degree in business administration or fields other than nursing may find they are not qualified to teach in any nursing program.

Although smaller private schools may be more likely to hire faculty who hold terminal degrees from for-profit organizations, larger private schools and public universities will be less likely to do so. *Where* you earn your terminal degree does matter. Even if administrators at larger schools have hired faculty with doctoral degrees from for-profit schools in the past, often once a "critical mass" of such faculty has been reached, hiring will be more focused on those with PhDs in nursing from research-intensive universities.

Those advanced practice nurses or nurse administrators who hold a PhD may be more likely to be considered for a faculty position than nurse educators who have chosen a DNP as their terminal degree rather than a PhD. Those advanced practice nurses or nurse administrators who hold a DNP degree may be more likely to be considered for a faculty position than those faculty applicants who hold a master's degree in nursing education and then chose the DNP as their terminal degree. The American Association of Critical-Care Nurses (AACN) recognizes the PhD as the preferred degree for nurse educators. A PhD in nursing from a research-intensive university may also be more highly valued and desirable than a PhD from a non-research-intensive university or from a for-profit university, and having a PhD in nursing from a research-intensive university may also qualify for a higher pay scale. You should seriously consider how wide of a net you hope to cast in job considerations prior to choosing a doctoral program. Do not choose a program that may simply be more convenient for you. Choose a program that is going to give you the most career-advancement opportunities.

FACULTY SCHOLARSHIP

Earlier in this chapter, questions were proposed about university support for faculty research and professional development. In addition to these, explore the SON resources and support systems for these endeavors.

■ THE PUBLIC UNIVERSITY PERSPECTIVE

Are students involved in faculty projects? Do faculty across disciplines collaborate on projects or teaching? Does the SON provide grants to faculty? Is there a nursing research office or access to statisticians and librarians? Does the SON purchase computer software for qualitative or quantitative analysis? The value and importance you place on doing research or engaging in scholarly activity will determine whether the university and SON you are exploring will meet your needs.

■ THE FOR-PROFIT UNIVERSITY PERSPECTIVE

The budget in for-profits is very closely aligned with tuition, so the money available for faculty scholarship varies considerably. You should ask whether scholarship is required and to what extent it is supported. Is there a certain amount allotted per individual or is there a pot of money doled out at the dean/director's discretion? Is the scholarship money targeted to improving oneself as a teacher or can it be used to pursue other professional interests? For-profit organizations require faculty development in accordance with their accrediting body's requirements. This development is typically focused on becoming a better teacher. Large organizations may have leadership development programs of which faculty can take advantage as well as ongoing coaching/mentorship programs for those already in leadership positions. Look in the faculty handbook (if one exists) to determine expectations toward scholarship and service. Most institutions in the sector do not engage in or support faculty research activities on the same scale as larger public or private universities. This is consistent with their career-focused mission and does not mean that they are not data driven. On the contrary, most institutions rely heavily on "dashboards" of data to make decisions at all levels of the organization. You should ask whether there is an institutional effectiveness/research department and how that department works with faculty to achieve desired outcomes.

■ THE PRIVATE UNIVERSITY PERSPECTIVE

Faculty scholarship at private organizations can be directly related to a number of factors. For example, faculty at research-intensive private organizations would have significant scholarship expectations. Faculty at small private universities may have lesser (or even no) expectations for scholarship. When evaluating potential teaching opportunities, ask specifically what the scholarship expectations are, and what support there is for scholarship. Support can include professional development, statistician support, grants, and other support.

It is this author's belief that all faculty members have the obligation to the profession and to the students they teach to engage in some level of scholarship. This might be in the form of original research, evidence-based practice, quality-improvement projects, or other forms of scholarly inquiry. Many faculty may choose to give up practicing nursing once they take on a position in academe, unless they are advanced practice nurses who maintain their certifications and must have a specific number of practice hours to do so. Giving up clinical nursing can significantly impact one's connection with "real-life practice." One way to stay connected is to conduct scholarship that is related to nursing practice. Leaders at healthcare organizations will often welcome a faculty member to assist with scholarly inquiry at their organizations. Ask about such opportunities.

COMMITTEE WORK

The faculty role may require committee work. During your interview, try to determine the expectations.

■ THE PUBLIC UNIVERSITY PERSPECTIVE

Your mentor should guide you regarding how many SON and university committees to involve yourself in and tenure and promotion expectations will also be informative in this regard. Saying no is probably one of the most difficult tasks for faculty, especially when new and eager to prove themselves a member of the team. Ask about the expectations and, once on the job, work with your mentor to learn when it is appropriate to say no to avoid overload.

What kinds of committees are standard at the university and the SON? On which committees might the nurse leader be expected to serve? What is the committee structure? You may find this in the bylaws. Does everyone get an equal opportunity to participate? To vote? If not, why not? Is there a small base of power within the SON that controls most of what is required and accomplished? Do tenure-track and adjunct faculty feel disenfranchised because tenured faculty are empowered to influence their success by withholding tenure or reappointment? These are nuances that may only be discoverable by talking to staff privately and attempting to guarantee confidentiality. However, people may be very reluctant to talk for risk of jeopardizing their standing. See Box 2.5 for examples of public university SON committees. However, committee structures can vary significantly from SON to SON.

Box 2.5 Public University: Examples of SON Committees

- Curriculum committee
- Undergraduate program committee
- Graduate program committee
- Academic standards or appeals committee
- Personnel committee
- Promotion and tenure committee
- Search and screen committee
- Evaluation or quality improvement committee
- Ad hoc committees

SON, school of nursing.

■ THE FOR-PROFIT UNIVERSITY PERSPECTIVE

Committee work will fall to the full-time faculty, who are few in number in most for-profit settings. Large multistate organizations are likely to have several levels of committee work and may assign workload credit for participating in committees at national or regional levels. Ask about workload credits for committee participation. Some institutions will pay for time spent in committee work, others will not. Organizations with many campuses will likely have centralized committees that may or may not have local representation. All will have at the least, admission and progression committees. Ask about curriculum and policy committees. Is there an honor society or other student committee that requires faculty oversight?

■ THE PRIVATE UNIVERSITY PERSPECTIVE

Committee work at private organizations is much like that described for public institutions. New faculty members are often allowed to take the first year to get acclimated to the faculty role without the additional burden of committee work. Committees may have criteria for its members based on rank and school. Most committees are such that there is equal and adequate representation from all schools.

APPLYING FOR THE POSITION

Chapter 3 presents information about applying and interviewing for nursing leadership positions so that information will not be repeated here. However, there are some distinct differences between applying for a faculty position and applying for a leadership position. The rest of this section will address these differences.

■ THE PUBLIC UNIVERSITY PERSPECTIVE

As stated in Chapter 3, the university may or may not employ a search firm. In any case, they will most likely have an SSC. Read the posted announcement carefully. Does your background match the required expertise? Consider the practical (or impractical) aspects of the job search. Applications and well-written cover letters are time-consuming and you must be prepared to respond quickly to SSC requests even though the committee or search firm may take its time responding to you. As you prepare to embark on a search, consider the following (Perlmutter, 2016a):

- Prepare mentally for a period of change and confusion
- Prepare logistically
- Keep track and update often
- Clear your calendar of extracurriculars
- Be ready to drop everything at a moment's notice

Once you decide to pursue an academic position or one different from the one you have, you must commit yourself to focusing on the search and the process. Be organized and systematic. Prepare a generic cover letter that you can alter to specifically address the expectations of each individual position. Update your cover letter and CV to include any new publications, conferences, awards, and so on. Keep your own database of universities to which you are applying, when or if you submitted your materials, what is missing, deadlines, and points of contact. Make notes about aspects of each SON or contact so you do not make the mistake of saying the wrong thing to anyone because you forgot details of your previous conversations.

■ THE FOR-PROFIT UNIVERSITY PERSPECTIVE

The for-profit university is an excellent choice for someone looking to start in a faculty role, since for-profits are interested in practical experience, not teaching experience, scholarship, or research. Certainly, candidates with richer backgrounds are preferred but all are welcome to apply. Most for-profits will consider applicants even if they do not have the desired credential. This is because, given the shortage of faculty, many nursing boards will grant waivers for faculty members who are otherwise qualified. For example, if a nurse with 15 years of experience as a pediatric nurse lacks the MSN, a waiver or exemption may be granted for a limited amount of time. This is especially true if the candidate is pursuing the desired degree.

■ THE PRIVATE UNIVERSITY PERSPECTIVE

First of all, potential applicants should read the position description and the desired qualifications carefully. If an applicant does not have the qualifications required or desired, that should be addressed in the cover letter, noting reasons why an applicant believes he or she should be considered anyway. For example, if a doctoral degree is required, but the applicant is near completion of a doctoral program or has recently been accepted to a doctoral program, explain that. Otherwise, if the application materials list the master's degree as the highest degree with no further explanation, the application likely will not be considered.

MAKING THE DECISION

■ THE PUBLIC UNIVERSITY PERSPECTIVE

Drive around the campus, the town, and the neighborhoods. Can you see yourself living here? There is more to life than work. Can you be happy here? Is there enough to satisfy your senses and give you the much-needed breaks that a stressful job requires? Think about the commute and parking. Is there a reliable transit system? Who pays for parking? The cost for parking in some metropolitan areas can be $50 a month or more. Include this factor in your salary negotiations. You may want to test the commute at the time you are required to be there and see what that is like.

Regardless of your assessment based on the interview, immediately send a handwritten mailed thank-you note to the chair of the SSC and possibly to those in higher administration with whom you met. Email is not sufficient. A handwritten note is more personal and shows that you took the time to write it to the individual. If you no longer want to be considered for the position, at minimum send an email to the search firm point of contact and the chair of the SSC.

■ THE FOR-PROFIT UNIVERSITY PERSPECTIVE

All considerations hold true for the for-profit sector a well. However, as there is no contract in these universities, ask about turnover, courses available for you to teach, how long the orientation is, and, if you are considering relocating, will they provide a stipend while you look for a home?

Given the uncertainty of the position, it is wise not to move the family or purchase a home until you have completed your first term. I am aware of a campus dean who relocated her family only to have her job category eliminated within her first 3 months of employment. Although of course this is the exception and not the rule, I have seen it happen several times.

■ THE PRIVATE UNIVERSITY PERSPECTIVE

Private colleges may often have a certain prestige associated them and a unique esprit de corps that is ingrained in students, faculty, and staff. With the higher tuition that students pay sometimes comes a greater expectation or assumption of success. Therefore, learn the policies for student acceptance and progression and the practices associated with them. This author has found parents to be much more involved in their children's private college experience than she saw in public universities. This does not necessarily equate with how much tuition costs, but could be associated with a connection to the mission or passion for the organization. This author sees a great pride in parents who are alumni of the private school who now have children attending the same school. That sense of prestige in attending the private school is handed down generation to generation. Faculty must buy in to the prestige concept and not see this as a distracting factor.

If deciding to accept a position at a private organization, wholeheartedly accept the mission and be prepared to be a role model for it. Part of the faculty contract may be to agree to abide by rules that align with the mission, even related to classroom topics. For example, at a Catholic or Lutheran organization, having a class discussion about abortion would be acceptable, but actively promoting a proabortion stance under any circumstance would not be acceptable under any circumstance. At this author's organization, a faculty member invited a guest speaker to discuss an abortion she had years earlier and how it impacted her life. She was not proabortion at all in her presentation. However, the faculty member did notify and receive permission from upper administration for this speaker prior to having her come to campus. If accepting a position at a private organization, a faculty member must be willing to abide by the set standards and rules that may be in place.

STARTING THE JOB

■ THE PUBLIC UNIVERSITY PERSPECTIVE

New faculty (and not so new faculty) often find the work of an academic to be overwhelming and unending. Contrary to what the public might think, faculty do not sit in their tweed jackets by the fire smoking pipes and expounding on the wonders of the universe. Faculty, in general, and nursing faculty, in particular, work extremely hard. Not only do nursing faculty teach but they also stay current clinically (one hopes), conduct research, publish, and present their work. Settling into a new faculty role can be intimidating and very exciting. It is helpful to understand that academe is very different from the clinical world. The organizational structure and expectations are very different but no less rewarding.

Krebs (2016) suggests new faculty "know the rules of the game." As mentioned earlier in this chapter and in Chapter 3, learn the policies and procedures of the SON, including how meetings are run and who gets to speak and vote and when. Per Krebs, the mentor should be the first stop for questions and then your direct supervisor: "You go to your mentor for advice and your chair [or supervisor] for permission."

Try to learn the formal and informal alliances within your SON and department. "Do not take sides—not yet, anyway. Be the questioner, the learner. Allow your colleagues to explain the issues to you from different sides—and don't stop at two" (Krebs, 2016, p. A44).

Strive to become an excellent teacher or improve if you are an experienced teacher. Serve on committees and be generous with assisting students and colleagues. These efforts will make your work life more pleasant and endear you to your colleagues and staff. As Krebs recommends:

> Go slowly. Try not to be guided by gossip . . . about who's toxic and who's not. Try not to become associated with a faction. . . . Form friendships with a wide range of folks, especially from outside the department [and SON]. Keep it professional . . . no matter how much your colleagues talk about being a "family." . . . Don't rush to make your place—let it evolve. (p. A44)

Watkins (2013) asserts that the first 90 days of your transition are critical to your success and suggests that during this time you learn the culture of the organization, develop horizontal relationships, manage vertical expectations, and refrain from "going in with the answer" but rather take time to learn and be open to new ideas.

■ THE FOR-PROFIT UNIVERSITY PERSPECTIVE

For-profit organizations are more likely to take a business-sector approach to onboarding and orienting. This is likely to be structured to acquaint you with all departments, both academic and operational. Do not underestimate the importance of the operations team to your own success. For example, full-time faculty in the for-profit sector work very closely with admissions and student services. You are likely to be observed teaching within your first 30 days. Take the time to have a thorough discussion with your director about that initial evaluation and areas to focus on. Remember, you are not under contract and can be released at any point. Most organizations are willing to work with you if you are willing to be the best you can be. In fact, for-profit institutions are accustomed to hiring novice teachers, so there is an inherent tolerance for "rookie mistakes." This makes the for-profit sector an excellent place to begin your teaching career.

■ THE PRIVATE UNIVERSITY PERSPECTIVE

When starting a new job at a private school, carefully remember the mission and foundational tenets of the organization. Starting a new job means being a novice again, and that can be frustrating and even daunting at times. Take time to learn who you can trust, never disparage others or take sides, and keep an open mind at all times. Listen more than you speak in the first few weeks and months. It can be especially comforting if other new faculty are starting at the organization at the same time, so you have confidantes within a cohort who are all experiencing the same new beginning, but this is often not the case. If you are at a faith-based organization, attend church or chapel services. Be sure you have a mentor assigned to you. There are pros and cons to having a mentor outside of the SON, as noted in Table 2.1.

Table 2.1   Pros and Cons to Having a Mentor Within or Outside of the SON

SON	Pros	Cons
Mentor within the SON	Familiar with SON culture	May be biased related to SON issues; on one side or other of issues
	Knows policies and unwritten rules	May advertently or inadvertently coerce you into a side or "camp" within the SON
		May advertently or inadvertently break confidence leading to bias from other faculty members

(*continued*)

Table 2.1   Pros and Cons to Having a Mentor Within or Outside of the SON (*continued*)

SON	Pros	Cons
Mentor outside of the SON	Neutral; not on one side or the other on SON issues	May not be able to provide sound advice on SON-specific issues
	Will be familiar with university policies and procedures	Will not be familiar with SON policies, procedures
	Confidentiality may be more certain	

SON, school of nursing.

Ideally, faculty members should look for a mentor within the SON and someone external to the SON but still within the university.

Starting a position in academe is very exciting. As a nurse you can influence people for whom you care; as an educator you can influence all the people for whom your students care throughout their careers. The influence is exponential. It is very rewarding to educate and mold the next generation of nurses, and it is a job that must be taken very seriously.

REFERENCES

Krebs, P. (2016, October 21). A guide to your new department. *Chronicle of Higher Education*, p. A44.

Perlmutter, D. (2016a, January 29). Academic job hunts from hell: Timing is everything. *Chronicle of Higher Education*, pp. A26–A27.

Perlmutter, D. (2016b, November 4). Do you fit us? *Chronicle of Higher Education*, pp. A22–A23.

Watkins, M. (2013). *The first ninety days: Proven strategies for getting up to speed faster and smarter*. Boston, MA: Harvard Business Review Press.

APPLYING FOR/SEEKING A NURSING LEADERSHIP POSITION

There are many different types of leadership roles in nursing academe. Nursing faculty who aspire to leadership roles, particularly associate deans and deans or department directors or chairs, should carefully consider what they are looking for beyond satisfying their ambition. These roles typically require more than 40 hours of work per week. Indeed, most require full-time responsibilities that go beyond the normal work week. Others, such as director or chair roles, might consist of half time in the leadership role and half time in the faculty role. In some universities, particularly in the public system, one may lose faculty status and, subsequently, the right to vote on faculty issues if the leadership role is designated for more than 0.5 FTE (full-time equivalent). The day-to-day workload rarely fits into the half time allotted for the position so it is very possible to teach 0.5 FTE but perform work required by the leadership role closer to three quarters of the time. You are correct that these do not add up to a 1.0 FTE and that is exactly the point! Associate deans and deans are typically designated as 1.0 FTE with the possibility of teaching a class on occasion. Consequently, director and chair roles are typically faculty with administrative responsibilities and associate deans and deans are administrators who may teach. Frequently, administrators are not permitted to vote in school of nursing (SON) committees or in university faculty committees. This chapter provides a broad examination of how you might approach researching and then pursuing a leadership role in nursing academe. Unless otherwise stated, the recommendations herein apply to all of the leadership roles thus far discussed; however, readers are encouraged to be selective as appropriate to the university or college in which they plan to seek a leadership position.

■ THE PUBLIC UNIVERSITY PERSPECTIVE

Although public systems of higher education share many similarities, they differ with regard to policies and procedures that may be unique to the system. Aspiring academic leaders must concern themselves with these policies because they are likely to play a role in enforcing them. Public systems tend to have many policies and processes that can cover almost any imaginable situation. Many policies are developed and maintained by the faculty and others are mandated by a Board of Regents or senior administrators from throughout the system who work together to standardize policies. Aspiring academic leaders seeking a position in a public university should attempt to learn about policies and procedures that impact the practices of the university and ultimately the SON. One can either locate these regulations on the system website or ask those within the SON how to find them. Review the system, university, and SON policies. They may differ but university and SON policies cannot be inconsistent with system policies.

If you want to be a transformative leader, you will want to work in a university that supports shared governance (Box 3.1). It is helpful to understand the degree to which there is shared governance in the university system. *Shared governance* refers to the degree to which faculty have a say in what happens within the system or university. Does the university to which you are considering applying have a faculty senate or council and do representatives from the senate or council represent the university at system meetings? How much say do faculty have within the university? Ask others how productive the faculty senate or council is. Do they tend to lag in getting anything done or do they listen to their constituents and move things along? Are the roles faculty play in governance likely to impede or assist the administration of the SON? What role do faculty members play in hiring decisions?

Shared governance can be helpful to the academic leader by providing the perspectives of all levels of the university; however, it may also

Box 3.1 Shared Governance

- How does the university define *shared governance* or do they call it something else?
- To what degree are faculty involved in decision making at the university?
- As an academic leader, will the degree of shared governance interfere with your ability to make decisions or enhance your ability to be transparent and transformative?
- Is there a faculty senate (made up of representatives) or do all faculty participate in the university faculty committee?

be somewhat of a hindrance if the academic leader must consult shared governance groups before making any final decisions. It may be difficult to get a true sense of how the system works until you are employed at the institution but be aware that this is a basic tenet of most public institutions and that, as an academic leader, you may have to operate within its confines.

The faculty senate or council is likely to play a role in approving tenure, promotion, and posttenure policies. Review these policies before interviewing for a leadership position, if possible. To what degree is the chair or dean involved in the promotion and tenure processes? This will give you a clue as to the influence of the faculty senate and to the degree of latitude you will have as a leader in making recommendations about promotion and tenure to the provost or president.

Managing or overseeing the budget is a primary responsibility of academic leaders, especially chairs and deans. What kind of model does the university use? Is it historical, incremental, activity based, or another type? As a chair or dean, you may have a significant role in managing the budget so you will need to understand it well. The budget model for the university may differ from the budget model used within the SON. For example, the university may use an activity-based model and the SON may use a historical budget. See Chapter 8 for a lengthy discussion about academic budgeting.

Aspiring nurse academic leaders will want to know the direction of the system, university, and SON (Box 3.2). How recently were the strategic plans reviewed and updated? Are the strategic plans for the SON, university, and system consistent with one another? You may not be able to access this information from websites but it is worthwhile asking whether you can review them as you plan for your interview. If you are invited to campus for an in-person interview, the SON strategic plan is a good starting point for discussing your vision for the school. It is very helpful

Box 3.2   The Direction of the System, University, and SON

- Strategic plans
- Websites
- Student and faculty handbooks
- Faculty constitution
- System, university, and SON accreditations
- Primary initiatives
- SON master evaluation plan

SON, school of nursing.

to review the SON faculty and student handbooks if they are available. These also provide clues regarding curricula, expectations for students and faculty, and how well organized the SON has been.

What are the university and SON accreditation organizations and the status of approvals, especially from the board of nursing? Programs close to renewal dates or seeking initial approval or accreditation will lean heavily on those in leadership positions to accomplish those goals. It is wise to determine where the program is in its process and whether there is a team dedicated to accreditation or compliance.

Ask to read the most recent accreditation self-study report to learn more about the SON, it strengths, and areas for improvement. Frequently, the self-study report provides the clearest picture of how the SON is doing and how it fits within the context of the university and the community. Ask whether there were any noted deficiencies or recommendations during the last accreditation visit. See Chapter 9 for a more in-depth discussion of accreditations and approvals.

SON typically have a master evaluation plan. This is a plan that is supposed to account for the specific details involved in meeting accreditation requirements, nursing association survey requirements, university requirements, and state board of nursing requirements. Does the SON have one? When was it last updated? How detailed is it? Does any one person have the responsibility for ensuring it remains current and that everyone is using it? Are faculty and staff aware that it exists? Ask to see a copy and review it. At a minimum, it should include all of the standards and key elements required by the accrediting organization and action steps for meeting the requirements of each standard.

Take time to review the university website and delve beyond the attractive face pages that are designed to draw students, parents, and prospective faculty to the university. Look at whatever the university has allowed the public to see and the disclosure section, as this is where information that the university is required to post but does not necessarily want to publicize is posted. Are there a lot of activities going on at the campus? Are there visiting professors and international trips for students and faculty? Are you able to find the information you need easily?

What do the SON web pages look like? Are they easily navigable? Accredited SON are required to ensure accuracy and consistency of the web pages and other public documents. Many schools wait until accreditation is due to update these materials. If the initial SON web pages are difficult to navigate, that may or may not be a clue to the success of the SON. It may require you to dig deeper to glean the information you need about the SON.

Look at the credentials of the current or former chief nurse executive (CNE) (see Chapter 2). The chief nursing administrator might be a director or chair or could be a dean of the SON. Was she or he selected from the SON faculty? If so, it might be a challenge to break into a culture that is already well solidified. How do your background and skill set compare with hers or his?

Throughout the interview process, see whether you can determine why the current CNE or the person you hope to replace is leaving the position. Is it simply time for this person to retire or move onward in her or his career or have there been problems within the SON or the university that might be worth noting?

Any prospective academic leader should be careful to investigate the organizational structure of the university and the SON (see Chapter 1 for more on this). What kind of structure is it? Is it very hierarchical or more horizontal? It is also interesting to learn whether faculty engage in interprofessional education activities and whether faculty from schools/ colleges outside of the SON participate on SON committees. The perspective of these outside faculty members is invaluable and adds richness to discussions and decision making.

As an academic nurse leader, know your faculty. Time spent researching who are on faculty and what they bring to the SON is time well spent. How prepared are faculty to teach? Do they have trajectories of scholarship? What kind of scholarship? Are their publications recent and in peer-reviewed journals? What is the ratio of faculty to other instructional and noninstructional staff? What is the expertise of faculty? Are there notable nurses on faculty? Do faculty serve on professional nursing organizations, corporate boards, and community committees? If the information about faculty is incomplete or outdated, this may also be an indication that either faculty are not very productive or there is little time or resources available to keep this information current.

Public universities may have their own unique structures of instructional staff. For example, the University of Wisconsin system employs faculty (tenure track and tenured) and instructional academic staff (IAS) who are required to teach but have no requirements (in many cases) for service or scholarship. IAS pay is considerably less than that of faculty and they may have to work for several consecutive semesters to acquire voting rights. Faculty and IAS may work well together or the latter may feel undervalued and that they have less of a voice. There are universities that only have faculty and everyone else is a clinical instructor or staff. Learn the structure and to try to understand the formal and informal methods and rules regarding communication and participation. It is also helpful to learn whether there is a union or collective bargaining agreement in place so you can inform yourself about pertinent policies.

What is the governance structure within the SON? SON typically use bylaws to guide their governance. These bylaws may be delineated for each committee within the SON or be an overall set of rules that govern the work of the SON. Bylaws are typically strictly enforced as opposed to guidelines, which tend to be malleable. The best bylaws are fairly general, allowing for unforeseen eventualities especially as they may have to go through lengthy processes to be reviewed and approved before they can be used. For example, in some public universities, changes to individual school or college bylaws may require review by an ad hoc committee, review by a formalized SON committee, review by the full SON faculty, open hearings, review by a university faculty senate bylaws committee, and finally, approval by the university faculty senate. Consequently, it behooves the aspiring nurse leader to request to review the bylaws to get a sense of how restricting they may or may not be on nursing leadership. Bylaws may tie the hands of the nurse leader to the extent that relatively little can be done by the nurse leader without multiple approvals.

Regardless of whether they are public, private, or proprietary, most universities have policies. A few were discussed earlier; however, SON also have their own policies (Box 3.3). These, too, may undergo lengthy processes to get approval or make changes. Ask to review the faculty handbook to gain a deeper understanding of these policies. Ask about the process for changing and updating them. Check to see when they were last updated.

It may also be helpful to contact healthcare agencies in the area and to speak to directors of nursing or chief nursing officers. The author has

Box 3.3 Basics About the SON

- Organizational structure versus actual governance structure
- Bylaws
- Faculty: expertise, engagement in research/scholarship/clinical practice
- Use and definition of adjunct faculty
- SON policies
- Reputation in the community

SON, school of nursing.

found that this can help provide a community perspective regarding how the SON is viewed by the community and how likely clinical partners are to hire the graduates or find placements for the students.

Internal candidates, or faculty who have decided to apply for a leadership position within their SON, also need to weigh all of the preceding considerations because the administrator perspective regarding these aspects of academe is very different from that of faculty. Try to approach the areas outlined earlier and in this book as if you were new to the university and the SON so you can acquire an objective viewpoint. As an internal candidate, you may or may not have an advantage over external candidates. The university and SON may want a fresh perspective and to hire someone "without baggage." You may have to work even harder than an external candidate to transition from a faculty to administrator role and lead people who have been your peers.

Applying for the Position

Public universities may or may not use search firms to recruit nurse leaders. However, it is not unusual, in times of economic stress, for public universities to reserve some money to hire search firms for deans and higher administrators because they want to cast a wide net and attract the best and brightest. Read the advertisement carefully and if a search firm is listed, contact them to discuss the position. Search firms can be great advocates for both the candidate and the SON because it is in their best interest to find the right candidate so they will be paid and be rehired for a future search. This author has found that they can provide good advice and less varnished views of what is happening at the university and SON than does the SON search and screen committee (SSC). Initial questions to the search firm are usually well received as you consider whether to throw your hat in the ring, but once the search firm has arranged a time and date for a "conversation" by phone or Skype, recognize that the "conversation" is part of the interview process and what you say may be passed along to the search committee. SSCs review the candidates the search firm recommends to see whether they want to pursue further interaction with the candidate. If there is no search firm, then the candidate will most likely deal directly with the chair of the SSC.

When answering the advertisement, include all of the materials requested or an explanation as to why you are not including them now but will shortly. If you fail to pay attention to detail, it is unlikely that your candidacy will progress. Remember that any interaction you have with the SSC chair or members is part of the interview no matter how casual it may seem. The search firm or SSC will first review the submitted materials to see whether the application packet is complete. If not, it is not likely they will look at any of the materials. Once the file is complete, the SSC will evaluate the materials to see whether the candidate meets its required criteria and then whether the candidate meets the preferred criteria. If the candidate meets the required criteria and has solid references, the SSC may choose to interview the candidate by phone or electronic media. In most public universities, there is an Office of Equity and Affirmative Action that must follow the law and university policies very closely. Ultimately, this office has to approve the candidates who will receive phone interviews and the final roster of candidates to be brought to campus to make sure that every effort has been made to include people from diverse backgrounds.

Take time to develop the cover letter, especially when applying for a leadership position, particularly a dean position. This author mistakenly included a one-page cover letter with her application during her first foray in seeking leaderhip positions. After all, faculty are typically instructed to keep the cover letter to one page and highlight the most relevant and impressive segments of one's experience. This author found out through a very helpful search firm executive and former university president that dean position cover letters are expected to be lengthy and address one's experience associated with each and every desired trait as described in the position announcement. Cover letters should be business-like, professional and specific, and should entice the reader to examine the CV carefully. Do not allow the reader to guess whether you meet all of the desired qualifications. Instead include a few sentences addressing your qualifications as they pertain to each desired trait and provide examples. Readers can review the CV for confirmation and detail.

Consider whom to tell about your search. Even close friends and colleagues might accidentally "spill the beans" to someone who knows someone. Particularly if you are already in a leadership position, and are looking for the next level of administration, it can put you in a precarious position if your supervisor finds out you are pursuing other options. Even the most supportive supervisor may begin to feel threatened and may begin to remove some of your responsibilities in anticipation of your departure. A vindictive supervisor might actually jeopardize your chances of getting the new position by giving you a poor reference. It is best to keep your own counsel until you know that you have a good chance of getting the position and you feel compelled to give your supervisor sufficient notice that you may be leaving. When you do give notice, clearly outline your plans for assisting with a smooth transition. Not only is nursing academe a small world and this will speak well of you but also your advanced planning and candid attitude are likely to reassure your supervisor that you are leaving on professional, if not good, terms and they can count on you to help with the transition.

The Phone Interview

If asked to participate in a phone or an electronic interview, first and foremost, listen to the question and answer it. If it is not offered, ask how many questions there are and how much time you will have to answer them so you can plan how long your answers should be. This author has observed candidates who spent most of their interview time on one or two questions and then did not have time to complete the interview questions. Too much embellishment, especially without actually responding to the question that was asked, is also a problem. SSCs tend to be composed of people selected because they will be working directly with the candidate or have expertise to understand who would make the best person for the job. SSCs see through attempts to skirt the question. It is better to admit that you do not have experience in a particular area but have a plan to learn about it than to avoid the issue at hand. SSCs understand that no one can be perfect or have experience with everything, but honesty and a willingness to learn are valued.

Make sure your technology works. For a phone interview, use a landline in a quiet private room. Do not use a cell phone as you drive along the highway. Clear reception is vital. A phone does not allow one to observe the nonverbal communication of the other party. Therefore, listen until the interviewer completes her or his statement or question, absolutely avoid interrupting, and be respectful and patient at all times. If the interview is to be conducted using a medium that allows all parties to see one another, then dress professionally. Make sure the room or office in which you will be sitting is clear of clutter and anything that might be distracting to the interviewers. You want the attention to be on you and not on your location. Ensure that it is a quiet room and that there will be no interruptions. Be very sure there is high quality and clear reception.

Visiting the Campus

If you pass the off-campus interview, then the next step may be an on-campus interview or there may be an intermediary interview that occurs near but not on campus. The search firm or chair of the SSC will help you with the details and make sure your trip and lodgings are reimbursed. Clarify information about who will make the arrangements and how you are to handle the receipts. Set your alarm to have plenty of time for unforeseen problems so that nothing interferes with showing up early for your interview. Fifteen minutes early is appropriate. You should be no earlier and no later. Try to get a good night's sleep before the interviews begin because there may be 1 to 3 days of interviews with minimal time to yourself. Eat a good breakfast so your belly does not grumble and you are less likely to be hungry later. Interviews conducted during mealtimes do not allow much opportunity for eating. Consider *every* interaction to be part of the interview, no matter how informal. Everything you do and say will be considered. If taken to a meal, avoid drinking alcohol unless you can sip a little without risking sounding or looking unprofessional. Do not order an appetizer or dessert although these will be offered. They cost more and public universities have minimal funding for these visits.

You will be given the list of interviews in advance. Prepare for each one. Bring a notebook with lists of questions for each person who will be interviewing you and wait until the time for questions (typically toward the end of the time allotted) to ask your questions. Questions are expected so make sure you have some. Also, make a list of your attributes that might apply to concerns each of the interviewers might have about your candidacy. For example, before you meet with the provost, do your homework and find out what you can about him or her. Make a list of what you might have to offer that align with his or her interests and priorities. You will be working for the provost so you will each be assessing each other for how well you can work together. It is perfectly acceptable to take notes but try to maintain eye contact as much as possible. If you have a sense of humor, use it, but strictly avoid jokes or comments that might give offense.

Do not disparage your current or former employer or university. This is considered in poor taste. If you are leaving or have left your previous employer because of something that you could not abide, then discuss the issue without laying blame on people. Not only are those people not present to defend their side of the story but academe is a small world, especially in nursing, and one never knows whom others may know. Remember that your visit to campus gives you the opportunity to evaluate the campus, the SON, and the environment as much as others are evaluating you. Can you see yourself in this role, working with these people? As a nurse academic leader there are things you will be able to change, but, much like a marriage, it is naïve to assume that you can change the fundamental way people think or act. Look at the classrooms, the labs, and the simulation equipment. Make sure there is an opportunity to meet with students without administrators or faculty and ask what they think of the SON, the faculty, and the university. They often have the most forthright and unvarnished opinions.

Making the Decision

Consider all of the points previously mentioned. If possible, speak to someone who is not on the SSC but who works or recently worked at the university or SON. Try to get as honest a picture of the position and environment as possible. Do not be rushed into a decision. If necessary, make another visit on your own with your partner or family to look around without the formality of the interview process. You will not be permitted the same access to places or information but you can get a sense of the environment. Observe people on campus, go into the student union, eat at a restaurant in town, and listen to the gossip.

Consider the position carefully. In many public universities, administrative roles are "at will," meaning you can leave or be fired at any time without cause or explanation. This can be an advantage to you but does not offer any job security. If the job is in an at-will state, does that position come with a faculty position and professorial rank? If so, then if something happens with your administrative role, you can revert to faculty and have job security until you decide on your next move. Taking an at-will position without this security is risky.

If you decide not to take the position, send an email to the search firm and/or SSC indicating your appreciation for the offer, that you enjoyed meeting everyone and having the opportunity to visit campus, but that you have decided that "this is not the best fit for you at this time." Be aware that SSCs often use the same language to let candidates know they have not been selected: "We regret to inform you that we do not think your experience or credentials are the best fit for us at this time." This is a lovely and professional way to indicate that your candidacy was not successful without citing deficiencies or hurting anyone's feelings.

Negotiating

Evaluate what is most important to you about this new opportunity. What is on your "make or break the deal" list and on what can you compromise? Sometimes the simplest things can be of the most importance, such as total reimbursement for your move and one to two trips to go house hunting. Many universities are willing to consider partner opportunities, but may not offer this unless you ask. For example, perhaps your partner is also a professor. Will the university also consider giving him or her a job without having to go through a search process? If this is not possible, can anyone at the university help pave the way for your partner to gain entry to new opportunities in the community or in the university system?

Some deans use the opportunity to negotiate to ask for new or additional faculty lines or an increase in budget for the SON. It is helpful to find out what the SON really needs and see whether you can work this into your negotiation. Regarding salary, the American Association of Colleges of Nursing (AACN) annual booklet *Salaries of Instructional and Administrative Nursing Faculty in Baccalaureate and Graduate Programs in Nursing* is extremely helpful in determining what the average salary is in the region and type of university in which you are interested.

■ THE FOR-PROFIT UNIVERSITY PERSPECTIVE

Much of what has been discussed with regard to public universities holds true for for-profit colleges and universities. However, consider the differences, especially if you are moving into the for-profit sector to take a leadership position (as opposed to moving up to a leadership position within the organization).

The most important difference is ownership. Some for-profits are owned by publicly traded corporations that have to satisfy the financial needs of the stockholders. This frequently results in setting leadership goals that are focused on enrollment and retention rather than the quality of the education. This is more likely to be true if the program is nationally accredited rather than regionally accredited, as the outcome measures for national accreditors focus on retention and placement. Corporate organizations also tend to be hierarchical, with standardized curricula, structure, and processes, so the leadership position may be strictly administrative with very little opportunity to influence curriculum or policies at the campus level. However, multicampus corporate programs do offer the opportunity to advance from campus leadership to regional and national leadership positions. You should be certain that you understand the nature of decision making that is both required and allowed, as well as opportunities for advancement before accepting a position with one of these programs.

On the other hand, many for-profit organizations are owned by individuals or families and have a very flat structure, with all decision making resting with the nurse leader. Although this may sound appealing, *all* really does mean *all*. The program lead is expected to recruit students and faculty, market the program, meet compliance regulations for the program and the university, oversee and develop programs, manage the budget, and, in some cases, do the payroll and other human resource functions. There may or may not be an expectation for teaching, but the responsibility for covering classes rests with the program lead and you may be pressed into service if an instructor is absent or you were unable to find faculty for all courses offered. There is more opportunity for creating and influencing the program in a flatter structure but there tends to be fewer resources, including faculty and support personnel. Family or privately owned programs may also have more risk associated with them, in terms of termination, especially in "at-will" states and in programs that do not offer contractual employment agreements.

Accreditation differs between the two types of institutions. Investigate who the accrediting agency is, especially if the agency is a national accreditor. National accreditation was historically given to career colleges and trade schools, hence the focus on retention and placement. Schools that have regional accreditation (most large universities) are often reluctant to accept credits from nationally accredited programs because of this difference in focus. This could interfere with meeting the deliverables assigned to the leadership position as well as the outcomes that must be met in order to be approved by the board of nursing or the nursing accreditation agencies such as the Commission on Collegiate Nursing Education (CCNE).

Securing appropriately qualified faculty is a responsibility of the nurse leader. This is challenging at for-profits that primarily hire adjunct or "visiting" faculty who have no ties or allegiance to the school and are probably working for many schools at the same time. A typical ratio for the for-profits is 60% to 70% adjunct faculty. The challenge is compounded by the fact that most for-profit programs operate 8- to 10-week terms. Therefore, the program leader should maintain good relationships with all faculty members to minimize turnover. You cannot just be pleasant and fair, you have to work at this in a very intentional way. One advantage of working within this type of program is the ability to make changes in the faculty with an ease and agility not found in public universities. Of course the disadvantage is that there is the potential for the nurse leader to be constantly "hiring," which takes energy away from developing the faculty. The number of full-time faculty varies with the number of students enrolled in the program and can be as few as three for programs of less than 100 students and as many as twelve for programs with 400 students. Small numbers impact decision making and committee involvement. Ask how faculty positions are allotted and how workload is determined.

Applying for the Job

The search process in the for-profit sector is similar to that found in public universities and usually starts with a screening phone call. Applicants with experience in the for-profit sector are preferred but not required. If you are new to the sector, having knowledge about the sector and how it is alike and different from traditional programs and understanding the mission of the organization to which you are applying will serve you well. Table 3.1 presents some of those differences.

There will be a number of interviews with a variety of departments outside of academics, including finance, marketing, and maybe even with the director of human resources. Unlike public programs, the faculty will

Table 3.1   Differences Between Traditional and For-Profit Programs

Characteristic	For-Profit	Traditional
Mission	Career focused	Education focused
Accreditation	National	Regional
Organizational structure/ oversight	Flat or matrix/board/of directors/stock holders	Bureaucracy/board of directors
Faculty governance structure	Limited within organization, but strong within program	Strong; usually a faculty senate or council
Class size	Small	Small or large
Funding	Tuition based and investors	Variety of sources, including donors and grants
Full time/ adjunct ratio	Approximately 40/60	Approximately 60/40
Academic calendar	8- to 10-week terms, no breaks	12- to 15-week terms with summer break
Admission starts	Rolling admissions with four or five start dates	Once or twice per year
Student body	Majority are part time, nontraditional; majority have credits from previous colleges or universities	Majority are full time; first time in college

not have input into the hiring decision. Be prepared to answer questions about retention, placement, budget, and operations in general, especially if the school only offers nursing programs as the campus leader is very often in charge of both operations (admissions, information technology, student services, etc.) and academics. Be alert to questions about your experience in getting accredited or obtaining board approval. Exploring your experience with these processes may indicate that the program is up for review. Ask about the program's accreditation and board of nursing status and what kind of support is available. You may want to contact the state board of nursing to determine whether there are complaints or issues with the program. You might also be able to find this information on the program's website under "disclosures."

Making the Decision

Before making any hiring decision, you need to be clear about your long-term and short-term goals. If you are interested in a research track, getting grant funding, publishing, or expanding as an academic, the for-profit sector may not be the right choice. Many federal grants are not available to for-profits. In addition, some publishing companies are biased against the for-profit sector due to recent negative press. Negative attitudes about the for-profit sector are changing, especially if the program has regional accreditation, but you should be aware that these attitudes exist and could impact future employment. If, however, you are interested in being a hands-on administrator with the opportunity to influence nursing education in very practical ways and collaborating with state and local leaders who have the same interests, the for-profit sector is the perfect place for you.

■ THE PRIVATE UNIVERSITY PERSPECTIVE

Faculty members seek leadership positions for a variety of reasons, including the desire to have more influence within an organization or within the profession, enhancing one's professional trajectory, and increased salary. Within clinical practice, promotions are often awarded to those who are good nurses. Within academe, promotions may be awarded to those who are good faculty members. However, without appropriate preparation for an administrative role, success can be elusive. Skills and abilities necessary to be a successful leader are different, although complementary, to those skills necessary for success at the faculty level.

Those aspiring to leadership positions should seek out professional development opportunities, such as the Leadership in Academic Nursing

Program (LANP) or the Wharton Executive Leadership Program, offered through the AACN. These programs allow participants to self-reflect on their leadership styles, hone and strengthen qualities necessary to lead organizations, and build knowledge and skills to manage relationships, influence people, and lead change.

Seeking a nursing leadership position within academe may involve moving into an administrative role within the current organization or looking for a leadership opportunity at another institution of higher learning. These pros and cons are summarized in Table 3.2.

When seeking an administrative position at a private college, in addition to reviewing all the documents noted earlier (bylaws, strategic plan, handbooks, etc.), thoroughly explore the foundational tenets or values of the organization. Leaders in a private university are expected not only to uphold these values individually, but also to promote these values and beliefs among peers, faculty, staff, and students. A leader in a private organization must be a continual role model both within and outside the organization 24 hours a day/7 days a week. The administrative leader becomes the face of the SON and one's actions are expected to align with the university and the school's mission, vision, and values. If the institution is faith-based, a foundational understanding of the religion is critical. It is not typically necessary to be a practicing member of that faith, but being a practicing member of a congregation in which the beliefs align and are not contradictory may be critical.

Potential applicants for a leadership position should have a basic understanding of how higher education is funded. Public universities are heavily supported through state funding, which is the main reason tuition is cheaper at public universities for students who are residents of that state. Private universities, on the other hand, do not receive support from state funds, but rather are funded primarily through tuition dollars, endowments, and donations from various sources. At private universities, strong enrollment management is critical because of the heavy reliance on tuition dollars to support operating costs. Students at both public and private institutions are eligible for financial aid. Many private universities offer substantial scholarship aid, and the cost to students and their families to attend a private university is usually well below the published tuition (sticker) price. Because private colleges are funded through sources other than state aid, their budgets are not reliant on the typical legislative state budget cycle, which can be heavily impacted by which party controls the Senate, House, and governor's office.

Because private universities rely heavily on endowments and donations, fund-raising skills and relationship building will be key elements

Table 3.2 Pros and Cons to Leadership Decisions

Leadership Decisions	Pros	Cons
Advancing within an organization	Understand organizational culture, policies, and procedures	Have established relationships that could interfere with leading
	Familiar with programs offered and their curricula	Others within the organization have preconceived ideas related to your leadership abilities based on prior track record
	Geographic move not likely necessary	Salary negotiations may be influenced by current salary
Taking a leadership position at a new institution	No established personal or professional relationships	Beginning at square one; must learn about faculty, staff, curriculum, university culture, SON culture
	Bring a new set of eyes to critically review policies, procedures, programmatic offerings, and the curricula	New ideas may not be perceived favorably by those embedded in the current culture
		Geographic move is likely
Moving from a public to private institution	Able to openly practice the foundational tenets of the organization	Faculty and staff salaries may be less than in public institutions
	Organizations can have fewer layers of bureaucracy	

SON, school of nursing.

of the administrative role for leaders within these organizations. Specifics on this are addressed in Chapter 4, but if applying for a role within a private organization, potential applicants should be aware that friend-raising and fund-raising will likely be an area that will explored during the interview process. When investigating a private university, applicants may want to seek out information on size of the current endowment and compare it to other private organizations of like size and in the same geographic location. Endowments may contribute to the university's operating revenue, so having a very small endowment could mean there is even more reliance on a steady enrollment from year to year to support operating costs. Small endowments may also indicate that alumni or community relations are not as strong as they could be.

Salaries for faculty and administrative leaders at private institutions may be less that they are for comparable positions within public universities. Unlike public universities, where faculty and administrative salaries are publicly available online or in libraries across the state, that is not the case at private institutions. If applicants are working with a search firm, discuss the potential salary range for the position and the applicant's salary expectations. It is a waste of time, energy, and money to apply and interview for a position if the salary range is not acceptable.

Applying for the Position

Private organizations that are faith-based organizations are allowed to ask applicants about religious preference and to hire selectively based on faith. According to the U.S. Equal Employment Opportunity Commission (EEOC)

> Religious corporations, associations, educational institutions, or societies are exempt from the federal laws that EEOC enforces when it comes to the employment of individuals based on their particular religion. In other words, an employer whose purpose and character is primarily religious is permitted to lean towards hiring persons of the same religion. This exception relieves religious organizations only from the ban on employment discrimination based on religion. It does not exempt such organizations from employing individuals due to their race, gender, national origin, disability, color, and/or age. (n.d.).

Those used to working at public institutions may be initially surprised when asked on the application for the name of the applicant's religion, parish, pastor, or other aspects related to the private organization's underlying foundation. Some private faith-based organizations have established policies regarding the percentage of faculty or administrators who must be practicing members of the faith. Ask about this, especially if not affiliated with the faith.

In a faith-based organization, if the faith is not one practiced by an applicant, and familiarity is weak, it is critical to obtain reliable and valid information about the faith to ensure those values are compatible with personal beliefs. For example, this author was raised and practices the Catholic faith. When a dean position opened at Lutheran University with an excellent reputation for its SON, reviewing the Lutheran faith was critical. It is not enough to "google" and look for information. Meeting with friends, family, or coworkers who practice the faith is a good way to explore issues and ensure that the values are personally compatible. For example, some faiths promote homosexuality as a sin, and condoning it would go against the tenets of the faith. Similarly, living with a partner outside of marriage may be enough reason to not be considered for a position if that situation violates the foundational beliefs of the organization.

It is impossible to "pretend" or to assume that an applicant can "pass" with limited knowledge of the faith, as many who work at private organizations are extremely committed to their religion, values, and other foundational aspects critical to the organization. Anyone seeking to be a "pretender" will be discovered very quickly. Applicants must come to terms with their individual ability to abide by those beliefs and uphold policies related to those beliefs if applying for a position within the organization.

At faith-based institutions, there are typically expectations to infuse faith in learning. Service also becomes synonymous with learning. Leaders at these organizations will be expected not only to comply personally with these expectations, but to enforce them with faculty and staff.

Box 3.4 illustrates common ways in which faith may be infused with learning or be part of performance expectations at faith-based private organizations.

Box 3.4   Infusing Faith at Faith-Based Organizations

- Prayer or devotion is used to open meetings
- Prayer used during class (before a test is common)
- Prayer used as part of student counseling and advising
- Teaching evaluations will include effectiveness on integrating faith in learning
- Performance evaluations will include mission in action

Policies at faith-based organizations will reflect the tenets of the faith. Some universities have a break for chapel, mass, or prayer each day. At this author's university, there is chapel break each morning for 20 minutes, during which time no classes meet and no meetings are scheduled. One semester, a new faculty member was assigned to teach a class in which the class "voted" that they wanted to opt out of chapel break. Rather than have class from 8:00 to 9:30, then chapel break, then resuming class from 9:50 to 10:30, the class voted to have class from 8:00 to 10:10 and "learn through chapel." However, the chapel-break policy is nonnegotiable, and this author had to discuss and reinforce the policy with the faculty member, who conveyed this to students. Although this decision may not have contributed to that student group's satisfaction, changing class time to conflict with chapel was nonnegotiable. Even meetings are not to be scheduled during chapel break. Whether faculty, staff, and students attend chapel or not is up to them, but they need to have the ability to freely go without the constraints of other scheduled business.

At private universities there may be celebrations commemorating key events associated with the history of the university or events associated with the mission. Days of service may replace class days. Losing a day of lecture or clinical may be well worth the opportunity to truly involve internal and external stakeholders in an event celebrating a momentous day or anniversary associated with the school or its mission. Leaders at private schools must not only support such events, but also be active proponents and participants, and this has to be considered when applying for a leadership position.

The Phone Interview

If invited for a phone interview, applicants can expect that questions will focus not only on the skills and abilities necessary for the leadership position and its expectations, but also on the fit with the mission of the organization. Interviews at a faith-based organization may start with a word of prayer or devotion. If the initial phone screening reveals concerns about the applicant's understanding of the organization, or the ability to uphold the mission and values of the organization, the applicant will likely not be considered further. So applicants should prepare well for the phone screening. If an applicant currently works in a public institution and is not accustomed to readily revealing underlying beliefs, rehearse this before the interview. Although questions may not directly focus on the organization's underlying mission or foundational tenets, it is a good idea to try to infuse those aspects into responses. This demonstrates an applicant's commitment and values as they align with the organization's mission. Other guidelines for preparing and participating in the phone interview for a private organization are like those detailed previously for public and proprietary universities.

Visiting the Campus

The on-campus interview is the next step in the process of securing a leadership position. For a faith-based organization, the interview day may include attending a religious service. If this is the case, it is interesting to note the numbers of faculty, staff, and students who are in attendance. This gives applicants a sense of faculty, staff, and students' commitment to their personal beliefs that align with the organization. If the visit falls around the time of midterm exams or finals, church attendance often increases as students are looking for any help they can get. (Divine intervention is appreciated.) It is necessary to feel comfortable in this environment as attending church may be an expectation.

The on-campus visit will typically include giving a presentation, meeting with the search committee members, meeting with faculty and staff, and meeting with other administrative leaders. This part of the interview will focus more on the candidate's potential to be an academic and visionary leader for the school. Observe how groups interact with each other and whether communication seems open and transparent. Watching the dynamics of the groups with whom an applicant is meeting can tell much about the organizational culture. Although much of the campus interview process is similar to that already detailed, it is possible that alumni or significant friends of the school may be invited to participate. Considering the role an academic leader will have in fund-raising within a private organization, external stakeholders may be invited to evaluate the candidate's potential related to this aspect of the position.

At the interview, ask about mentorship and support that will be available should the applicant be offered the position. If applying for a dean position, typically a dean from another college or an academic vice president would be an excellent mentor. New deans need to have someone outside of their school with whom they can confide openly and honestly. At the interview, be watchful for someone with whom such a connection might seem reasonable. At a private university, an interview with a member of the Board of Regents or other governing body may be included to assure mission fit with the organization. At such an interview, there will be greater focus on the applicant's personal beliefs, values, and practices than on the skills and abilities related to academic leadership. Board of Regents' members assume that qualifications for the leadership role will be appropriately vetted by the faculty, staff, and administrators who have already interviewed the candidate. The role of the mission-fit interview is to assure the applicant's compatibility with, and ability to promote, the foundational tenets of the organization.

Ascertain exactly how much authority and responsibility the dean has within the SON. For example, ask questions about the organizational structure, workload, and budget. Come with a list prepared and if those questions do not get answered during the day as part of the interview, meet with the person who would be serving as the immediate supervisor to get clarification. Leave the interview with as much information as possible about the role and its responsibilities and expectations so that an informed decision can be made whether this is a good fit for both the applicant and the organization.

If the applicant has worked with a search firm, salary expectations have likely already been conveyed to organizational leaders. However, if a search firm was not involved, the applicant will want to discuss salary expectations openly and respectfully with the person responsible for making the salary decision for the position.

Making the Decision

If offered the position, the applicant needs to weigh all options before making a decision. If an applicant has gone through all the screening and has been offered the position, it is assumed that leaders and faculty within the organization are convinced of the applicant's leadership abilities as well as the mission fit. Similarly, an applicant has considered his or her leadership skills and fittingness within the organization before applying. However, an applicant must truly soul-search to ensure that the mission is consistent with personal beliefs as organizational values and tenets are at the core of everything from academics to the overall campus culture. To accept the position, one is confirming a readiness to embrace and model the mission, not only at work, but also during off hours as well. It will also mean a commitment to ensure that faculty, staff, and students similarly embrace the mission. Typically, this decision to accept or decline an offer cannot be made quickly, and the applicant is wise to take time to consider it carefully. However, the applicant should give the employer a timeline upon which a decision will be made.

Negotiating

If mission fit is confirmed, accepting the position involves negotiating a salary, workload, and academic rank upon entry. Salary expectations should have been discussed earlier, either with the search consultant or the person at the organization who will make this decision. The AACN annual *Salaries of Instructional and Administrative Nursing Faculty in*

Baccalaureate and Graduate Programs in Nursing includes salary data for private universities and this can be helpful in determining an appropriate salary for the geographic area and like-size private universities. One goal for salary is to be at least in the 50th to 75th percentile of the means of salaries for like organizations within the same geographic area. Being a new dean does not allow one to expect to be at the top of the salary range, but one does not want to start out in the lower half of the mean salaries either.

If teaching is part of an administrative load, negotiating a lighter teaching load (or no teaching responsibilities) for the first year is wise. This way a leader can immerse herself or himself fully in learning the administrative responsibilities without having to prep and teach class and be directly responsible to students for coursework.

Negotiate for the appropriate academic rank. For example, a person will want to ensure that academic rank in a new position equals or is higher than what is currently held, assuming that the person meets the qualifications for that academic rank at the school to which a move is being considered. Criteria for rank vary, so the applicant may have to be ready to defend his or her qualifications for a particular rank. If an applicant has service responsibilities, such as being a journal editor, member of a board, or other like positions, be sure that those activities will be supported and can be maintained in the new role. It is wise to get a written memorandum of understanding (MOU) to have documentation of what was agreed upon as part of accepting the position.

REFERENCE

U.S. Equal Employment Opportunity Commission. (n.d). Pre-employment inquiries and religious affiliation or beliefs. Retrieved from https://www .eeoc.gov/laws/practices/inquiries_religious.cfm

CHAPTER 4

FUND-RAISING/DEVELOPMENT

It is increasingly necessary for universities to seek donors and raise money. With decreases in state and federal funding, nursing faculty and administrators must look to the generosity of alumni and community partners to share their "time, talent, and treasure." Deans in public and private institutions especially have been asked to devote more of their time to fund-raising. Nursing education does not include a course in fund-raising. "Development" might be an excellent topic to include in nursing curricula in the future.

Nursing faculty and administrators typically have experience interacting with others, if not to solicit money, then as therapeutic communication or to teach. Nurses are inherently comfortable talking with strangers and developing a rapport quickly and effectively because of our experience with patients. This ability and experience puts us somewhat ahead of our nonnursing peers when we enter the world of fund-raising.

■ THE PUBLIC UNIVERSITY PERSPECTIVE

The view that higher education is for the public good has become controversial. As Nicholas B. Dirks, chancellor at the University of California at Berkeley, said, "It is increasingly clear that there are significant differences between university communities and state governments when it comes to the interpretation of 'public mission'" (2016, p. A56).

These differences often lead to reduced funding for public universities and an increasing need to rely on fund-raising to build and sustain programs.

Schools and colleges of nursing may or may not have designated development officers (DOs) who are professional fund-raisers. These are people who have often learned their trade through experience and at the feet of more experienced and successful fund-raisers. They often come to academe from the private or corporate sectors.

A good DO always knows his or her audience, knows how much and how long to woo prospective donors, and when to go in for "the ask." The DO should also have a good relationship with the chief nurse executive (CNE) in the school of nursing (SON) because the two must work together systematically and strategically. The DO might work with more than one college within the university and typically answers to a chief DO and a foundation office. The foundation is made up of a volunteer board that determines the strategy and goals for fund-raising. The foundation president is likely to be a corporate leader with many years of fund-raising experience. The board members are volunteers who typically have a degree of wealth that allows them to contribute heavily and frequently to the foundation. Otherwise, they may be invited to be on the board because they have a vast network of influential people or entrée into high society. The board is responsible for the management of the foundation funds.

Public universities are funded by taxpayer monies so this money is distributed based on strict rules. For example, public money cannot be used to fund foundation activities or projects. If you are in a leadership position, learn the rules so you do not inadvertently misuse public funds.

The Role of the DO

The DOs in the university solicit donations to the foundation but may or may not sit on the foundation board. A good DO is part visionary, part idealist, thinks and dreams big but also knows when to let it go and when another nudge or outright push will seal the deal. They must be well organized and stay abreast of what alumni might want and to what they are most likely to respond.

The DO arranges events, such as lunches or dinners, to include the prospective or current donor and the dean or CNE. He or she must also be part detective to try to determine who else the donor might like to see and whether students or faculty are the way to the donor's heart. Keep up with the life events (and deaths) of donors as a large portion of donor funding comes from estates and wills.

Prospective or current donors are often invited to homecoming and other university events. The university and SON might have competitive alumni awards and host a banquet to celebrate awardees. Electronic and paper newsletters and magazines are commonplace and serve to remind alumni and other friends of the SON that the SON is busy, active, and growing. These communications as well as others, such as emails or mailers, celebrating nurse's week and other important nursing events help the friends or prospective friends of the SON feel included. Selected stories about student and faculty accomplishments and innovations might just stimulate something meaningful to the friend and encourage him or her to donate to the college to help continue the good work.

The Role of the Nurse Academic Leader

The nurse academic leader plays a key role in seeking or identifying prospective donors and in cultivating them. For example, when this author began her role as dean, several alumni donors and other donors requested to meet with her, presumably to learn her vision for the SON and determine whether they still wanted to contribute to the future of the SON. These meetings were important and it was necessary to prepare for them. This author worked with her DO to learn details about each donor so that she could have conversations that were individualized to the interests and projects of the donor. It was also necessary to encapsulate her vision for the SON in a couple of brief statements that could be expanded if the donor sought further information.

One key to a productive conversation with a donor or prospective donor is to remember that the conversations and meetings are mostly about the donor. The nurse leader must be a good listener not only to be polite but to be alert to how the donor or prospective donor relates specifically to nursing. Is the donor a nurse? If not a nurse, has he or she or a family member been cared for by a nurse? If so, was it a good experience? The nurse leader must make the case that the SON is educating nurses who will be well prepared to care for patients and meet the needs of the donor. For example, perhaps the donor is an older adult. Then, direct the discussion about nursing education to how nursing students are being prepared to provide excellent care to older adults. In any case, emphasize your excitement about the future of nursing and the SON and how your vision will advance both. Avoid discussing specific financial needs at a first meeting unless asked.

It is probably unusual to have a situation like this author did with a donor who had been supporting the SON for a long time but whom the author was meeting for the first time. The author picked the donor up at the hotel to take her to an event. No sooner were they both in the car, then the donor turned to the author and said, "So, what do you need?"

Some donors are very frank and ask what they can do to support the SON. Deans and faculty should always have an answer ready, the famous "elevator speech." *Elevator speech* is the common term for a very short (30 seconds or less) story one might be able to tell in the course of a typical elevator ride. For example, you are riding an elevator and someone notices that you are wearing a sweater with the name of your SON printed on it. Your riding companion says something like, "Oh, do you work at so and so school of nursing?" You do not simply answer yes and mind your own business. You launch into your elevator speech in which you very quickly highlight all of the wonderful things happening at the SON and how excited you are about them. You might then say, "Here is my card. I would love to meet with you some time and tell you more about what we are doing." If you feel comfortable, ask the person about himself or herself and see whether they will provide you with a business card or contact information.

Prospective donors can be found behind every corner if you are alert to the possibility. The grocery store is a likely place. Academic leaders may be easily recognizable by people in the community so be aware of possibilities through the activities in which you are involved, outside of work. Someone on your faculty or among your staff might sit on a community board or have friends and neighbors who do. These connections can help you learn of the goals and priorities of foundations and prospective donors. You and your DO can then develop a plan that aligns with those goals and priorities that could lead to a future donation.

Once the DO, academic leader, or others have identified a prospect, everything should go through the DO. The DO will have to check with his or her colleagues at the university to make sure this prospect is "not taken" by another DO. The DO may then reach out and make the first contact, which might be a meal with the academic nurse leader, if the prospect is local. Otherwise, the DO might encourage the nurse leader to send a note to the prospect highlighting something that might be important to the prospect or worthy of note about the SON. For example, DOs might see something in a newspaper, alumni publication, or social media and suggest the nurse leader send the prospect a note congratulating him or her or expressing interest in the activity or event. This opens a line of communication that the DO will monitor. The DO can then advise the nurse leader about the next opportunity to make contact. Several contacts are typically required before the DO feels it is the right time to ask for a donation or "feel out" the prospect for the likelihood of a donation.

Biemiller (2016, p. A9) describes a five-step approach, called *moves management* that includes identifying potential donors, finding information about them, gauging their interests, getting them involved, and persuading them to invest. The nurse leader may also want to assemble an advisory board or council made up of carefully selected donors who are invested in the success of the college. This group might meet once each semester or as necessary to help with fund-raising efforts. Members should be kept to a small number but selected based on their history with the college, past record of giving, and time and ability to assist with SON fund-raising. Typically, the members will donate a certain amount per year as part of their commitment to being on the council. Keep members apprised of what is happening in the SON and make them feel valued and respected. Others should be made aware of their participation and importance.

A document that outlines the mission of the advisory council and the responsibilities of the members is helpful for all involved. It should make clear that the objective is to assist the college with fund-raising and should delineate how and when meetings are held. If a donation is required, then that should also be clear.

An annual fund-raising event can be very effective. The advisory council can be tasked with putting it together and hosting the event. Also, events, such as SON anniversaries or other occasions, can be reasons to stage an event that draws current and potential donors and alumni.

The CNE in the SON is frequently the highest paid or, at least is assumed to be by faculty and staff. Not only is contributing a personal donation the right thing to do to support your school but it sets an example to those with whom you work and prospective donors that you also believe in the causes you are espousing and you "put your money where your mouth is."

Donations or gifts can start at any level and all are valuable. Frequently, small donations lead to larger donations and it is the relationship that is key here. Planned giving and estate planning are cornerstones of successful fund-raising. Nurses may have a particular advantage in this respect as people with chronic illness or who have had nursing care over the years may not need much encouragement to include an SON in their estate planning.

The Role of Faculty and Staff

All faculty and staff should be provided with the basics of fund-raising because one never knows when one might encounter someone during or outside of university business who might be a prospective donor. Know what to say, when to say it, and to whom, as faculty and staff act as ambassadors for the SON.

This author has attended several workshops and has organized workshops for faculty to learn about development and fund-raising.

To accomplish it correctly and to avoid "putting one's foot in one's mouth" the dean, faculty, and staff should learn the SON's elevator speech and to recognize clues that someone might be worth cultivating as a potential donor.

Gone are the days when faculty and staff left fund-raising to the administrators and DOs. Funding for public universities is such that donations are necessary to build and renovate buildings, labs, and classrooms; purchase equipment and simulation manikins; provide student scholarships; help fund study abroad; and innovate. Faculty and staff are key players because they interact with students and visitors who may be encouraged to have an interest in donating.

Working With Foundations

According to Masterson (2016), while foundations vary, they frequently share similar aims: They want to have maximum effect, facilitate change and fund something meaningful. Foundations, unlike individuals, want to support an area of their interest. Individuals often give out of loyalty regardless of their interest.

Judith Shapiro, former provost and college president and current foundation president, offers words of advice on working with foundations (2016). She advises to attend meetings fully prepared to explain programs for which one wants support and with a thorough understanding of the foundation's mission and priorities. Foundation grants tend to be short term, but foundations want to know that their gift will keep on giving. In other words, one must make a case that the gift will fund a program or project that will be sustainable and have significant, long-term impact. Dr. Shapiro also emphasizes the need to "inspire confidence." The academic leaders who meet with foundation representatives should be ready and willing to share information about the university (and the SON) that align with the priorities of the foundation, but should also know how to present an interesting idea without appearing self-aggrandizing or self-promoting. Masterson (2016) suggests a checklist to consider when working with foundations (Box 4.1).

Box 4.1 Public University: Working With Foundations

- Assign one person to work with the foundation
- Be strategic
- Consider each foundation unique with unique interests

(continued)

Box 4.1 Public University: Working With Foundations (*continued*)

- Invite foundation representatives to campus and carefully prepare for the visit
- Present data-based ideas that are new and interesting to that particular foundation
- Offer opportunities to collaborate
- Remain in touch with the foundation whether or not you receive the grant

■ THE FOR-PROFIT UNIVERSITY PERSPECTIVE

For-profit schools are owned by individuals, families, or investors. Funding comes through private investments or the sale of stock. Therefore, there are no expectations for raising funds other than actively marketing the program to attract students. For-profit schools and universities rely heavily on Title IV student loans and Pell grants. So much so that Section 487(d)(4) of the Higher Education Act (HEA) of 1965 requires for-profit schools to submit a report annually regarding the amount and percentage of the institution's revenues from Title IV sources and non-Title IV sources recorded in their audited financial statements. Title IV funds include the loans and grants listed in Table 4.1.

More than half of the nearly 2,000 proprietary schools in the United States reported receiving greater than 80% of revenues from federal loans and grants in the 2014/2015 academic year (Federal Student Aid, U.S. Department of Education, 2016). By law, for-profits must meet the 90/10 rule, which stipulates that for-profit schools must be able to demonstrate that at least 10% of revenues come from sources other than these federal programs. This 10% usually comes from self-paying students or those accessing their military benefits provided by the GI bill. For-profits aggressively advertise and market their programs, which has resulted in increased scrutiny from the Department of Education. This increased scrutiny has led to new levels of transparency in the sector, which ultimately has the potential to attract students who are a good fit for the program and will persist to graduation. According to Deming, Golden, and Katz (2012), for-profits spent approximately $4,000 per student on recruitment efforts in 2011 with almost 24% of revenue invested in sales and marketing efforts. In addition, all faculty and staff are expected to market programs and recruit students by providing services to the surrounding community, visiting military bases, visiting high schools, and attending open houses.

Table 4.1   Title IV Loans and Grants

Direct loans	Largest provider of Title IV funds. These loans can be subsidized or unsubsidized based on financial need. Students can receive up to $12,500.00 per year.
Perkins loans	Loans made by the college or university. Students with exceptional need can receive up to $5,500.00 per year.
Pell grants	Loans for undergraduate students who do not have a bachelor's degree. The amount awarded is based on need and cost of attending and varies annually. The maximum amount for the 2016/2017 academic year was $5,815.00.
Academic competitiveness grant	Designated for first- and second-year college students who qualify for Pell grants who are attending school full time and have demonstrated academic ability. The award for first-year students is $750.00 and for second-year students is $1,300.00.
National SMART grant	Available for third- and fourth-year college students who are eligible for Pell grants and who choose to study physical, life, or computer sciences; math; technology; or engineering. The maximum award is $4,000.00.
Federal Supplemental Educational Opportunity Grants	Campus-based funds that are not available at all campuses. Varying amounts of money can be awarded up to $4,000.00.
Federal work–study	Funds provided to support student employment.

SMART, Science and Mathematics Access to Retain Talent.
Source: Federal Student Aid, U.S. Department of Education (2017, February 26). *Federal student loans: Basics for students.* Retrieved from https://studentaid.gov

Student clubs and organizations can and do participate in fund-raising activities to support student events or scholarships. These activities range from bake sales to raffles. Care must be taken when raffling expensive items since there are restrictions on the amount of money for-profit organizations can accept in the form of contributions. There are also state and local ordinances that must be adhered to.

Although some for-profit schools have alumni associations, they are usually not well organized and do not have fund-raising as their mission. The purpose of the majority of alumni associations is to mentor current students and provide networking opportunities for graduates. Of course, like their not-for-profit counterparts, for-profit public relations and marketing departments enjoy highlighting the accomplishments of graduates to raise public awareness and attract more interest in their programs.

■ THE PRIVATE UNIVERSITY PERSPECTIVE

As noted in Chapter 3, private universities rely heavily on endowments and donations because they do not receive financial assistance from the state as public universities do. Therefore, academic leaders, as well as faculty and staff, will be called upon to actively and continually participate in friend-raising and fund-raising activities. Although the academic leader typically works closely with the DO, faculty and staff also play key roles in identifying potential donors whose goals and passions align with the SON, as well as meeting with those who may share an interest with the faculty or staff members' particular expertise or initiatives. It is critical to cast a wide net for potential donors whose interests may align with those of the SON.

Fund-raising is based on relationships. Nurse leaders should look at every encounter as a potential for a new relationship. New relationships can take 2 to 3 years to cultivate to become "comfortable." Established relationships need to be continually nurtured in order for them to grow and flourish. If a good and trusting relationship is established with open communication related to the activities within the school, often the DO or academic leader may never even have to do "the ask." Potential donors will feel so connected to the SON and its initiatives, they will offer support before it is even requested.

In the past, large healthcare organizations were often key contributors to support schools of nursing, their infrastructure, and their activities, because the products of the school (the nurse graduates) are critical to the function and success of the healthcare organization. However, as healthcare organizations struggle with narrowed profit margins that go along with greater public and private demand to reduce costs, healthcare organizations have a decreased potential to donate large sums of money. They are also heavily invested in the local communities in which they serve, and tend to spread their donations to a wide variety of projects that benefit the community as a whole. When supporting SON or other health professions, leaders within healthcare organizations often want to "stay neutral" in that they must support the vast network of SON and other health professions with whom they collaborate. Thus, they may be less likely to give to one, because they are very unlikely to be able to give equally to all.

Healthcare organizations are themselves recipients of generous donations for a variety of their own projects and initiatives. Leaders within healthcare organizations may be reluctant to give to private schools for fear of alienating others (their donors, employees, or customers) whose beliefs may not align with the private school's mission. These are issues that need to be openly explored and discussed among DOs, academic leaders, and leaders within healthcare organizations when looking at the potential for donations and other support.

It is critical to identify potential donors who align with or have a passion for the activities, mission, or goals of the SON, and who have the same alignment and passion for the private school's foundational tenets. Of course, alumni would typically fit this pool because they chose the school to receive their education. Therefore, nurturing potential donors begins with the student experience. Academic leaders should look upon each current student as a potential future donor. It is critical to establish an esprit de corps among students that fosters loyalty, connection, enthusiasm, and passion for their school. The intent is for those feelings of loyalty and connection with the SON to continue after graduation. Private schools that have a strong service component are also establishing a sense of "giving back" with their students that can be fostered and nurtured with the hopes that it will continue after graduation.

New graduates often begin careers dealing with student debt (which can be higher if they attended a private school) while they are establishing themselves in the community in which they have gained employment. They may be renting their first apartment, buying their first home, buying a reliable car, getting engaged and married, and starting a family, all of which take a considerable amount of money. Therefore, relationships with alumni may not result in donations for at least the first 5 or even 10 years as alumni get their financial health established. Academic leaders need to recognize that continuing relationships with alumni are critical so that when their earning power is greater and financial health is stronger, alumni will remember their connection with the school and choose to allocate donations. New graduates make excellent tutors or mentors for current students. Having graduates return to discuss their experiences studying for and taking the NCLEX® exam, getting their first job, or guest lecturing on a topic connects them with the school and with current students. Having alumni involved with school activities does not have to cost them anything during a time when they may not have the means to make a monetary donation. Keeping them involved keeps them connected, and kindles the relationships with the school and its leaders, faculty, and staff that could foster the potential for future donations.

Larger private schools and those that graduate alumni who have greater earning power (doctors, lawyers, business leaders) may have an easier time garnering larger donations from their alumni. At smaller private schools, a greater number of alumni may be working as teachers, social workers, life coaches, or in other professions that do not earn significant incomes. Yet these are groups with a strong sense of community and service. They touch the lives of many others through their work. The people they touch may be willing to donate to the school in which the teacher, social worker, or life coach was educated.

Nurses tend to make very good salaries and have great potential to give back. Nurse leaders should look to nurture that sense of giving and sacrifice that is often present in those who choose nursing as a career. In addition, nurses touch a tremendous number of people in their work, and it is possible that nurses' impact on patients and families could create a sense of philanthropy in those whom they touch. Nurses heal, accompany patients through health and illness, save lives, and assist with birth and death, all momentous events that could trigger those impacted to donate to the school in which the nurse was educated. That esprit de corps, if properly established while in nursing school, will follow nurses who will proudly share where they learned their craft and received their education.

All nurses understand the difficulty of going through nursing school. Many nursing students must work to maintain health insurance and to support living expenses while in school. Appealing to nursing alumni to contribute to scholarships to assist current students is often met positively. Alumni will donate so that perhaps current students can work less and study more. Like parents wishing for a better life for their children, nurses often wish for an easier path through school for nursing students and will contribute to scholarship funds. Alumni know the academic rigor of the nursing curriculum and they realize that each year there is more to learn as healthcare gets more and more complex.

Each donation, no matter how big or small, should be recognized, preferably with a personal note of thanks. This author has asked to be notified of each gift to the SON so that she can write a personal thank-you. One can never thank a donor enough. If thank-you notes come from the DO and the nursing leader, those are welcome recognitions of one's gift. The size of the gift does not matter, as even a small gift may just be a "sample" of what may come later. A gift of $10 could turn into something much greater in the future if the generosity of the donor is recognized and valued.

Alumni often donate to "be a part of it" with the "it" being whatever moves them to write a check or establish an endowment to support the school. For example, when larger private schools, such as Marquette University or Notre Dame, are featured on national television playing basketball or football, alumni (and others) can be moved to donate to feel they are a "part of it." Smaller private schools may have to work harder to gain and maintain widespread visibility among potential donors. Newsletters, newspaper articles, social media reports, and other updates may help to showcase the school and its activities when television coverage is not an option. Featuring alumni and their accomplishments in newsletters is a key way to rekindle the esprit de corps that was established during their education. Recognizing alumni publicly with some sort of award could lead to a donation back to the school. This author has been recognized by her high school as a member of the Alumni Hall of Fame and by the institution in which she earned her doctoral degree as a member of the 50 Distinguished Alumni. Both of these awards triggered donations to the schools.

With private schools, it is not reasonable to assume that all or even the majority of donors may be intimately connected with the mission. Reach out to those in the "public" world to let them know what is going on at your private school. Those not directly affiliated with the founding organization may be pleasantly surprised by the initiatives and activities that connect the school with the community, and their interest could spark a sense of giving.

With private organizations, it is possible that a decision must be made to turn down a donation if it comes from a person or organization whose foundational beliefs do not align with the school's mission. Although this can be a difficult decision, leaders at private organizations are used to the notion that mission is at the core of everything. Denying donations from organizations whose beliefs or practices are contrary to that of the school, is the ethically and morally correct decision.

Nursing leaders have to understand institutional priorities for fund-raising and work closely with the DO to support these. For example, when this author began her position, a new business building was set to break ground on the Wisconsin campus and fund-raising efforts were focused on that project. This author continued relationships with donors and potential donors, knowing that not all were interested in giving to the business building. However, in the grand scheme of things, a new nursing building would likely be "next in line" on the Wisconsin campus. Nursing leaders must realize that when the institution wins, everybody wins, and they must support all initiatives both publicly and privately, even if they are not directly connected to nursing. When supporting institutional priorities, they are supporting the campus that supports nursing. As noted earlier, it can take 2 to 3 years to establish and nurture a relationship. Therefore, potential donors to a nursing building that might be built a few years down the road can easily be cultivated for several years before a new nursing building takes shape.

Nurses are excellent relationship builders, and they also have assessment skills that allow them to "read" people in a way that many others do not. Therefore, fund-raising abilities often come easily. Because nursing is typically the most trusted profession, this fact reflects positively on potential donors, who can trust that their support will be valued and their donations will go to a very good cause. Nurses have the potential to move people in many ways; it is logical that they could also move people toward supporting a cause or initiative. The true efforts lie in determining each potential donor's passion or connection with the school, which will motivate them to lend support financially or in other ways.

Although DOs focus on fund-raising, some smaller private schools may have a mix of DOs and advancement officers (AOs). AOs do more than just fund-raising and sometimes one person may hold the role of both DO and AO. AOs may organize campus events like community breakfasts, leadership-development talks, presidential roundtables, or other such events that connect community leaders with the school. Community leaders are often honored to be featured speakers or to be a part of a panel discussion on a topic of interest. As noted earlier, nursing administrators should look at every encounter with a community member as a potential fund-raising opportunity. When AOs are planning events, nursing leaders should take an interest and be involved. Often nursing leaders are asked to provide names of key community members to whom event invitations should be extended. Any opportunity to bring a community member or community leader to campus is an opportunity to showcase school programs, initiatives, and activities. It is also an opportunity to showcase students who have a remarkable ability to pull at the heartstrings of potential donors. Students' accomplishments often can move donors to dig deep in their pockets to support education. So, although this chapter focuses on DOs and fund-raising particularly, readers should also be aware of the role of AOs and how they can also initiate activities that could trigger fund-raising opportunities.

Having the opportunity to showcase your SON and raise funds to support efforts within the school and to support students in their nursing education is truly a privilege. Nursing leaders need to take these opportunities seriously, and work collaboratively with DOs and AOs in order to establish ongoing and productive relationships with alumni and other key stakeholders.

REFERENCES

Biemiller, L. (2016, February 12). Presidents of small colleges bank on fund raising to survive. *Chronicle of Higher Education*, p. A9.

Deming, D., Golden, C., & Katz, L. (2012). The for-profit postsecondary school sector: Nimble critters or agile predators? *Journal of Economic Perspectives*, *26*(1), 139–164.

Dirks, N. B. (2016, July 22). Flagships must create new models to preserve the public good. *Chronicle of Higher Education*, p. A56.

Federal Student Aid, U.S. Department of Education. (2016). 90-10 attestation report AY2015. Retrieved from https://studentaid.ed.gov/sa/about/data-center/school/proprietary

Federal Student Aid, U.S. Department of Education. (2017, February 26). *Federal student loans: Basics for students*. Retrieved from https://studentaid.gov

Masterson, K. (2016, December 16). How to court a foundation. *Chronicle of Higher Education*, pp. A8–A9.

Shapiro, J. A. (2016). Foundation leader's advice: Come to the meeting prepared. *Chronicle of Higher Education*, p. A10.

CHAPTER 5

RECRUITING AND MANAGING QUALIFIED AND DIVERSE FACULTY AND STAFF

Recruiting and managing faculty and staff occupy a great deal of the time of nurse academic leaders. Recruiting faculty has become increasingly challenging in recent years. Public, private, and proprietary universities recognize the need for increased diversity of faculty, staff, and students. People from diverse backgrounds, including, but not limited to color, ethnicity, religion, culture, gender preference, and (dis)ability, bring different perspectives to the academic environment and thus help it move forward and continue to be relevant to an ever-changing society. They also more closely represent the students and patients we serve in our communities. Depending on the university and whether it is public, private, or for-profit, there may be more or less funding and other support for recruiting faculty, staff, and students. In addition, resources and rules may differ with regard to advertising and targeting of people from diverse backgrounds.

Managing faculty and staff requires finesse and knowing when and if to speak and what to say under very challenging conditions. Other books and resources go into leadership and management models and techniques in great detail. This chapter does not seek to, nor could it duplicate those in-depth resources. However, the authors share some tips and techniques that have worked for us, which cross all types of universities and schools of nursing (SON).

■ THE PUBLIC UNIVERSITY PERSPECTIVE

Before recruiting faculty and staff, the nurse academic leader must ensure that the funds exist to pay them. This may sound commonsensical; however, it is not enough to consider salary. In public systems, fringe benefits can be exorbitantly high, as much as 50%. You will be hiring based on current market prices so comparisons with veteran faculty and staff are not particularly helpful. In addition, salaries in public universities are visible to all so there may be employees who are angry or disappointed that newly hired faculty and staff have higher salaries than they do. If this is the case, you may be able to convince the university to allow you to raise salaries. However, you may not have the funds available to do so.

The American Association of Colleges of Nursing (AACN) issues an annual booklet that lists the aggregate salaries for faculty and administrators in nursing programs in public, secular, and religious schools and colleges of nursing, by region. These data provide a solid foundation from which to negotiate higher salaries for your current or prospective faculty.

Think about your goals for the SON. Are you hoping to attract faculty from out of state? Internationally? If so, then what salary would bring them to your SON? What other incentives might be meaningful to them? Are you seeking rich resources to support research and scholarship activities? Funding and other support to improve teaching and student success?

Develop a detailed and accurate position description. The human resources department can share examples that have been used throughout the university. However, this author has found it helpful to research what other similar SON have included in their position descriptions. What exactly does the SON require? In the case of faculty, consult your chairs or directors to determine the types of classes that need coverage. What are the expectations of research and scholarship? Are you willing to hire a new graduate or should the person already have a solid program of research or teaching experience? Do faculty teach clinicals? How much service in the SON, university, community, and profession is required? Are there other special responsibilities to include? Wording of position descriptions can be key to recruiting the faculty for whom you are searching. Take the time to carefully craft the description and the job announcement sent.

The staff with whom new staff will be working should be included in decisions about the characteristics needed and be on the search committee.

The support staff often set the tone within the offices. They greet visitors and students and work together closely to ensure the smooth working of the SON. The primary duties of the position should be clearly delineated in the position description, but that wonderful phrase "other duties as assigned" should always be included.

The university's mechanism for ensuring that all people, regardless of race or ethnicity, ability or disability are treated fairly may require that particular wording be included in the position descriptions. This is to be consistent with the law and to make it clear that, as a public university, there is no tolerance for discrimination. The office that handles this will probably provide this wording; however, it is good to participate in training, if it is offered, to learn what is permitted in position descriptions and in the hiring process.

Public universities tend to have complex processes for obtaining approvals to hire. The position description is only one part of that process. Find out the process your university uses and learn whether there is an electronic system for candidate applications.

The SON may or may not be expected to pay for advertising. Similarly, the SON may be expected to create its own advertisements or may have a university marketing department that can assist. Whether or not the funding for marketing and recruitment comes out of the SON budget or from a university central fund is also variable. Typical advertising venues include nursing newsletters and websites, professional conferences, and professional organizations such as the AACN. *The Chronicle of Higher Education* is also a very good resource.

In public universities where funds are limited, choices must be made to utilize scarce advertising and recruiting dollars. There is a certain expectation for advertising in journals that particularly target people of diverse backgrounds. Your university may present you with data to demonstrate how many people from diverse backgrounds you must hire in order to meet university requirements. Nursing may make the argument, as this author has, that there are relatively fewer numbers of men and minorities in nursing than females and nonminorities. Therefore, recruiting them is especially challenging. This does not excuse or absolve the SON from trying just as hard to recruit men and people from diverse backgrounds. It just helps university personnel to understand that the SON may need professional assistance to conduct a successful search.

Public universities will differ widely with regard to the proportion of faculty, staff, and students from diverse backgrounds. Those located in major cities may have many more people from whom to choose than rural universities. However, it may still be a struggle to recruit and hire people from diverse backgrounds because those hired must be qualified and because there is competition from other schools to hire the same qualified people. In addition, the search process "is often rife with personal biases, groupthink, power dynamics, rushed judgment, and potential conflicts of interest, while relying on imperfect measures of intelligence, experience and ability" (McMurtrie, 2016, p. A20). McMurtrie wrote of the liberal use of the term *fit* during college searches. That term is frequently used to describe why a person, for whatever reason, is not recommended for employment. Academe remains predominantly White despite the increased diversity of students on college campuses (McMurtrie, 2016).

The university is likely to have an office that manages equity and affirmative action issues. Title VII of the Civil Rights Act of 1964 prohibits discrimination in organizations of 25 or more employees. The office will have guidelines about hiring practices, particularly how to ensure that people from diverse backgrounds have had a fair chance to apply for the position. This office or the human resources office on campus may conduct training on implicit bias that can help faculty and administrators understand how their own subconscious views can negatively influence the search process.

Search firms can assist in faculty searches but they are costly and vary significantly in the services they provide. Public universities may have budget restrictions that preclude using search firms except in cases of higher administrative positions. Wilde and Finkelstein (2016) recommend that search committees analyze what they want from a search firm and how they will define a successful search. They suggest sending a request for proposals to selected search firms to invite them to apply. A rubric to evaluate each firm that applies can be helpful to determine which has the best price and services. Finally, legal counsel can be invaluable in developing the contract with the search firm.

McMurtrie (2016) recommends that universities plan in advance and not wait until they need to hire someone. Planning can lead to banks of potential recruits. Generally, openness to others and a concerted effort to introduce potential recruits and faculty and staff candidates to others on campus with whom they might work on topics of mutual interest can yield significant dividends.

Nursing has not always been open to nontraditional applicants whether they be ethnically or culturally diverse or different with regard to their educational or experiential backgrounds. We tend to think inside the box when it comes to deciding with whom we will work and who will teach our students. Nursing is trying very hard to increase opportunities for interprofessional education so it logically follows that we should more frequently consider faculty and staff from other cultures as well as disciplines when trying to broaden our students' horizons. Nursing has had study-abroad opportunities for a long time and many universities hire international faculty. However in nursing, this is more likely to happen in large universities and those with strong research agenda. A strategic plan for inclusivity within the SON that specifically states the goals and action steps the SON will take to increase diversity and inclusivity will help keep the SON on track in this pursuit. Outreach efforts, such as attending conferences specifically to search for diverse faculty and requiring a diversity statement in candidate applicant packets, can also help in this effort.

It is not enough to simply recruit and hire faculty from diverse backgrounds but to treat them fairly once they are employed. Patricia A. Matthew, an associate professor of English, wrote a book about the experiences of faculty with diverse backgrounds (as cited in Brown, 2016) describing how universities could ensure more equity. According to Matthews, "the goal is 'let's hire a person of color and bring them in to *diversify*' without a real understanding of what that means and how to value it" (p. A8).

Some universities hire diversity consultants to assist them with their planning (Schmidt, 2016). The focus on diversity and inclusivity cannot just be in pockets of university activities, such as recruitment. "True institutional commitment to diversity permeates every aspect of the campus and is widely collaborative" (Harper, 2016, p. A25). Goldrick-Rab (2016) suggests some specific strategies when committing to diversity (Box 5.1).

Managing Faculty

Managing faculty and staff requires patience and fortitude. Nurses who are still primarily focused on their own notoriety will be unsatisfied as academic leaders because the attention must be on others. The new academic leader or nurse assuming a director, chair, or dean position should take the time to meet with each individual within the SON, regardless of his or her role. The time spent can go a long way to resolving issues that arise later. If the academic leader has risen from within the SON, then these meetings can still be useful because they can be used to establish

Box 5.1   Strategies When Committing to Diversity

- Collaborate with the school district in your area, address disparities, and offer a welcoming environment.

- Use innovative approaches to intentionally recruit low-income people and those of color.

- Build relationships in the community and demonstrate openness in admissions and financial aid.

- Hire faculty, staff, and administrators of diverse backgrounds and hire from the community, when possible.

- Provide adequate support systems to meet the needs of students.

- Involve parents and families in college life.

- Honor alumni and encourage them to mentor and role model for students from diverse backgrounds (Goldrick-Rab, 2016).

the change in relationship. These meetings with individual faculty and staff should revolve around three questions: What has been working well, what has not been working well, what the individual's professional goals are, and how the academic leader can help support those goals? Having faculty and staff submit these in writing prior to the meeting can be helpful in guiding the discussion and also be filed for future reference. When issues or conflict do arise, and they will, reminding oneself of what's important to the individuals involved can be very helpful.

Many of the personnel issues that arise, at their core, simply require someone to listen and moderate the discussion so it stays on track and does not devolve into personal attacks. The biggest challenge to academic leaders, especially nurses (who are used to talking and intervening to solve problems) is to sit quietly and listen. The people working for us are typically smart and capable people and can work out their problems if given the opportunity to be heard.

It also behooves nurse academic leaders to stay in touch with their faculty and staff. Everyone becomes so busy that semesters pass before one can turn around. Create opportunities to stay connected beyond monthly faculty and staff meetings. Consider lunch opportunities, wherein a small group of faculty or staff lunch with the nurse leader privately. Sit in on faculty and staff meetings to just listen and be available to respond to concerns but arrange to do this in advance. It is not a good idea to make surprise visits unless there is an urgent message to deliver.

Be careful to keep your own counsel within the SON. In other words, it is not a good idea to confide too much in anyone and when you do confide, remember to whom you said what. Find someone outside of the SON with whom you can talk freely and ask for advice. AACN offers a dean's mentor program that connects new deans with experienced deans. This author has found this relationship to be invaluable.

■ THE FOR-PROFIT UNIVERSITY PERSPECTIVE

The manner in which faculty are recruited and hired varies with the type of institution. A large multicampus organization will likely have a centralized human resources department that recruits and screens all potential candidates before forwarding résumés to the local campus leadership. Smaller institutions may delegate that activity to the nurse leader who typically opens a job request in a human resources software system and checks periodically whether any candidates have applied. Human resources only gets involved when the hiring decision is made or when the job has gone unfilled for a prolonged amount of time. Most for-profits have their own search teams and rarely outsource recruitment. Unlike traditional programs where faculty search teams are involved in interviewing and vetting candidates, the faculty at for-profit schools may not be involved in the process at all. Schools that do involve faculty usually do so by having them participate in the candidate's teaching demonstration, which is a standard requirement for hiring didactic faculty and, in some places, for hiring clinical faculty as well.

Finding qualified faculty is increasingly challenging in all parts of the country. This is especially true for the for-profits that typically pay less and do not offer the security of contracts. Given that difficulty, most for-profits hire to fill vacancies without much regard to diversity. That is to say that they don't hire with a diversity mind-set. This is primarily because they hire local experts who are likely to represent the diversity in the community they serve so they end up with a diverse in makeup faculty and staff as a matter of course. In addition, the majority of faculty in the for-profit sector are adjuncts and adjunct pools tend to be the most diverse in makeup (Finkelstein, Conley, & Schuster, 2016). While finding qualified full-time faculty is challenging, the sector is fairly successful in hiring a qualified pool of adjunct faculty. This is due in part to the freedom and flexibility found in these institutions as a result of the shorter terms, the wide variety of assignments and locations, and lack of commitment for committees or outside activities. Diversity is rarely an issue in large metropolitan areas such as Washington, DC; New York; Detroit; Chicago; Baltimore; Los Angeles; and Boston. In fact, a study conducted by the Teachers Insurance and Annuity Association of America (TIAA) (Finkelstein et al., 2016) shows a significant increase in hiring minority faculty with a 11% decline in the number of White faculty overall. Note that diversity extends beyond consideration of race, to include people with disabilities, gender-identity issues, sexual orientation, and religious preferences. It is interesting to note that in academe in general, women are underrepresented among full-time and tenured faculty. The opposite is true in nursing faculty who are primarily female. In for-profits, as in other sectors, there is a desire to increase the number of male faculty members, but there is no specific recruiting effort targeting that population and, in most cases, the most qualified faculty member will be hired regardless of gender. We tend to hire people like ourselves, which creates an inherent bias when screening and interviewing. Having an awareness of this bias will increase the likelihood of creating a diverse faculty body. Additional practices to ensure a diverse faculty are listed in Box 5.2.

Box 5.2   Additional Practices to Ensure Diverse Faculty

- Look for nontraditional career paths or experiences
- Inquire about experiences with diverse student populations
- Look for involvement in service organizations
- Avoid the tendency to prefer those from elite colleges and universities

Flaherty (2016) contends that diversity goals will not be met until the minority groups in the adjunct pool move up to full-time and tenure-track positions. These positions are not available at most for-profit schools, so diversity is addressed by growing the "pipeline" or creating a pathway for students to become faculty. According to the National Center for Education Statistics (Snyder, de Brey, & Dillow, 2016), the number of minority students entering college is increasing across all ethnicities. Minority students are drawn to for-profit colleges because of the more relaxed admission requirements and flexible schedules. These students are future faculty and need to be encouraged to continue their education beyond the baccalaureate level. Faculty need to articulate the joys and benefits of teaching so graduates will want to join the ranks.

Managing faculty can be quite a challenge for the for-profit sector because very often the faculty are novice teachers and are not familiar with academic settings or expectations. They are often hired just before the term starts with little or no orientation to the faculty role. They are not required to attend meetings, and may not have any contact with other faculty or campus leadership. In addition, the adjunct may be teaching at several other schools at the same time that have different expectations and they may only teach for one term making follow through with development impossible. Some institutions do offer promotion in rank for full-time faculty. These institutions are able to set standards for instructional practices that foster consistency and best practices. Remember though, that full-time faculty are small in number in the for-profit sector. The wise nurse leader will focus on developing each faculty member by fostering their growth as educators, including curriculum development and classroom management. Assigning a mentor for adjunct faculty is also key to both developing and retaining a qualified pool of both classroom and clinical instructors. Strategies for managing and retaining faculty are listed in Box 5.3.

Box 5.3 Strategies for Managing and Retaining Faculty

- Discuss mission and values of school of nursing.
- Assign a mentor to assist with the technical aspects of the role such as using the learning management system, technologies in the classroom.
- Provide opportunities to observe or team teach with a "master instructor."
- Schedule "touch points" at least biweekly in the first 90 days.
- Observe in the classroom to offer both praise and opportunities for improvement.
- To the extent possible, let faculty select their courses for the next term well before the next term starts.

Managing Faculty

The organizational structure of for-profit organizations usually separates operations from academics and therefore the nurse leader may not be involved in hiring or managing staff. In some cases, administrative staff are shared among departments. When this is the case, expectations, reporting structures and priorities, should be clearly stated. When the nurse leader oversees both academics and operations, he or she will need to have a good understanding of the skills needed to be effective in admissions and student accounts. Managing these staff members also requires an understanding of federal regulations related to how their jobs are carried out. Tensions and resentments sometimes arise between staff and faculty when there is a perceived inequity in expectations related to attendance, work schedules, and perks. The best way to manage this is through transparent, open dialogue with the parties involved and making sure job roles and expectations are clear. When possible, operations staff and faculty offices/cubicles should be located in the same area, as this fosters collaboration and understanding. Pink (2011) asserts that what motivates people is the opportunity to control their own destiny, be creative, and have purpose. Finding ways for both faculty and staff to have these opportunities will increase retention and satisfaction.

■ THE PRIVATE UNIVERSITY PERSPECTIVE

As noted in other chapters, leaders within private universities put a significant amount of effort into recruiting faculty, staff, and administrators for mission fit at all levels within the organization. This can influence the focus when hiring diverse faculty and staff as the mission fit may limit diversity, even if the intent is not to do so. Faculty who apply at private organizations often do so because of their strong connection or belief in the mission. Leaders have to be sure that connection is not something that stifles diversity or "outside thinking." At this author's university, there are some faculty members who obtained their bachelor of science in nursing, master of science in nursing, and doctor of nursing practice all at this school because of their passion for the mission. They are proud of their three-time alumni status and are wonderful, dedicated faculty members who live the university's mission. Yet, they have never been exposed to alternate viewpoints, or to curriculum, policies, and procedures at other organizations. This can lead to entrenchment in "how things have always been done" or defending why things are done the way they are based on historical data that may no longer be relevant. Many universities will not hire doctoral students as faculty members immediately after graduation. Rather, leaders at these universities encourage graduates to go somewhere else for a time and then they may consider them for hire at a later time. This is done to promote diversity in thinking and to expose faculty to other schools' curriculum, policies, procedures, and research agenda, and to other faculty and administrators' ways of thinking.

Faith-based organizations can selectively hire based on religious preference, although they cannot discriminate. This author had a very capable colleague who retired from a public university, but since she was Hindu, hiring her as an adjunct professor at my faith-based organization was not possible. We require that all faculty and staff are Christian. The same is not true for students, where those of all faiths are welcomed, accepted, and supported. Even students who identify themselves as atheists are welcome. However, at a faith-based school, students will all be exposed to the mission and the faith of the organization. The underlying message is not to convert them, but simply to expose them to the faith.

Students at private universities tend to be more diverse than faculty. Private universities, especially smaller organizations, can have a significant number of diverse students who perhaps did not meet academic admission requirements at larger public universities. Some diverse students believe they will be more successful learning in the smaller classes and can be more engaged with faculty, which is what most private universities tout. Private universities often recruit heavily for international students, because the higher private school tuition is often very comparable to out-of-state tuition at public universities or tuition for international students. If certain countries are targeted for student recruitment, there can be a significant number of students from that geographic area. Therefore, they recruit diverse faculty and staff in private organizations to better reflect the diverse student body.

Students in higher education need to be exposed to diverse viewpoints in order to be better prepared for the challenges they will face in an increasingly diverse society when they graduate. A successful way to do this is for them to learn from diverse faculty. However, hiring diverse faculty has been an issue for several decades and the number of diverse faculty at both public and private organizations remains significantly less than their Caucasian counterparts. Diverse faculty typically represent only a very small minority of the faculty numbers overall (Taylor, Burgan Apprey, Hill, McGrann, & Wang, 2010). Smith (2009) and Lynch (2013) argue that a diverse student body alone is not enough to justify hiring diverse faculty. Diversity among faculty members will infuse diversity into the curricula, research, and strategic initiatives at the university. Diversity is self-supporting, meaning that attracting diverse faculty members will assist in attracting other diverse faculty members as well as in attracting diverse students. Being hired for faculty positions in some fields can be very competitive and diverse faculty may come up short in their in past teaching, research, and service experiences when compared to Caucasian applicants (Lynch, 2013). Yet, that seems to be less the case with nursing faculty positions, as the numbers of positions available are typically much greater in number than the numbers of qualified applicants. Nursing leaders have for years been trying to attract more diverse students and faculty to better meet the healthcare needs of our increasingly diverse society and to better teach diverse students.

When seeking diverse faculty members is a priority, academic leaders should carefully oversee and select members of the search committee who are committed to that same goal. Casting a wider net when advertising for the position may be critical especially if the university is located in a geographic region that may not be very diverse itself. Advertising in journals, on websites, and in organizations that attract diverse readers or have diverse members is important, especially when private universities are located in smaller communities as opposed to those that are in larger metropolitan areas. Ensuring the search committee is made up of diverse members will make a more favorable impression on a diverse applicant, and a first impression ensures that a potential candidate is not turned off early in the search process. Like public universities, private schools have a person or department that handles affirmative action matters and including someone familiar with affirmative action on the search committee is a good idea. If an affirmative action officer is not available to be a member of the search committee, committee members should ask whether there is affirmative action training to familiarize themselves with best practices for hiring diverse faculty and staff. Similarly, sometimes search committees may bring in a diverse community member who can assist with questions about the community fit and resources and to better explain how the diverse faculty or staff member may be welcomed into the community.

Because diverse faculty are highly sought and recruited, the lower salaries that private universities typically pay could be a stumbling block to hiring them. Academic and administrative leaders will have to determine what is the special determinant that might be appealing at their university that would entice a person of color or an underrepresented minority to take a position at the school. What is special about the school could be any number of things, including strong mentorship options, favorable teaching load, support for research, opportunities for global travel, a good match with the student population, or a strong connection to the school's mission. A higher salary might attract diverse faculty members, but if other nontangibles do not contribute to a welcoming culture, the salary alone will not be enough to retain them.

Although men are considered a minority in SON, and women are considered minorities in many science, technology, engineering, and math (STEM) fields, another minority in academe may be the younger generation. Generation Xers born 1966 to 1976, Generation Y (Millennials) born 1977 to 1994, and soon even those from Generation Z born 1995 to 2012 could technically be completing advanced degree programs and applying for positions as faculty members. Potential faculty members from all of these groups demand a better work–life balance than the baby boomers who currently dominate academe. Baby boomers tend to do whatever it takes to accomplish something, often at the expense of family, vacation, or free time. Generation Xers demand a sense of community, and Millennials tend to be more diverse themselves and have been exposed to a greater amount of diversity during their lifetimes (Trower, 2010). If search committees are dominated by aging baby boomers who may be turned off by the younger applicants who put a greater priority on free time and family before work, there may be problems recruiting younger faculty to replace a rapidly aging nursing faculty workforce. In addition, as baby boomers get farther and farther removed from the age of the students whom they are teaching, there can be a sense of disconnect. Therefore, younger faculty members can have a positive effect on the impressions that students and potential students have when coming for visit days or other student recruiting events. If all they see is faculty who look more like their grandparents, this could deter them from choosing the school for their nursing education.

Although I have used the term *faculty* primarily in this section, everything can apply to hiring diverse staff as well. Staff will not have the teaching, research, and service expectations that faculty have, but they will be continually exposed to the overall culture of the SON and the unit in which they work. Academic leaders have to ensure that culture welcomes and supports diversity. Staff (advisors, skills lab and simulation personnel, and administrative assistants) can also interact with students even more than faculty. Thus, hiring diverse staff members will better meet the needs of a diverse student body.

Managing Faculty

When diverse faculty members are hired, they can experience difficulty in adjusting to the culture that is dominated by a Caucasian majority. It is critical to understand that the hiring process is fairly easy when compared to retaining highly qualified diverse faculty members and ensuring they are satisfied in their role. All faculty should have a comprehensive orientation program, but especially diverse faculty who may not be familiar with academia or with aspects of the dominant culture in which they will be working. Providing diverse faculty with an opportunity to review and discuss university and school handbooks along with policies and procedures will assist them in getting acclimated to expectations. The discussion will allow questioning and clarification. If diverse faculty have English as a second language, jargon that is sometimes used in written handbooks may be confusing. Helping new faculty understand any "unwritten rules" that are part of the dominant culture will be critical to their success. This author had a colleague who once asked why she never knew about the unwritten rules until she had broken them.

Having an in-depth discussion about the private school's mission and any accompanying behavioral expectations should be clearly spelled out during orientation. One cannot assume that a diverse faculty member would know these expectations if they have not been immersed in a culture consistent with that of the private school. If a diverse faculty member has never taught before, expectations for faculty need to be addressed, not only in regard to teaching, scholarship, and service, but also for professional development in academe in general. A strong orientation program will be the foundation for positive socialization into the faculty role and can contribute to satisfaction and ultimate success.

Another aspect associated with success for new faculty members is a strong mentorship program that focuses on assisting the faculty member to achieve milestones necessary for promotion and/or tenure and other expectations for teaching, scholarship, and service. Faculty new to academe may need greater assistance with aspects of the faculty role and a trusted mentor can provide guidance in these areas. Some highlights for developing and a sustaining successful mentor/mentee relationship are included in Box 5.4. Some information applies only to teaching faculty, and some applies to all faculty and staff.

Box 5.4   Highlights for a Successful Mentorship Program

Teaching

- Guidance and feedback in developing course materials
- Assistance in developing evidence-based teaching strategies
- Classroom management
- Dealing with students
- Understanding how to use instructional technology
- Developing evidence-based assessment and evaluation strategies

Scholarship

- Accessing funds to support research
- Travel funds to support research dissemination
- Grant-writing opportunities
- Steps to successful dissemination (publishing and presenting)
- Acting as a peer reviewer for the mentee before manuscript submission
- Continuing education

(continued)

Box 5.4 Highlights for a Successful Mentorship Program (*continued*)

Service

- School and university committee work
- Community service
- Involvement in nursing professional organizations
- Service to the church at faith-based schools

Other

- Socialization to the faculty role
- Opportunities to practice nursing
- Global travel

The mentoring relationship may continue for a year or even longer, so the mentor and mentee should develop mutual goals for the relationship to familiarize themselves with expectations. Like a strong orientation program, a comprehensive mentorship program is associated with faculty retention and ultimate success in the faculty role.

University officials may engage community members as additional mentors to welcome new faculty members into the community. This may be even more helpful for international faculty and staff who may need assistance obtaining a driver's license, getting housing, setting up bank accounts, navigating the healthcare system, selecting schools for children, finding a place of worship, and other aspects related to everyday life.

If international faculty are hired, teaching nursing courses without a strong knowledge of the healthcare system in the United States and nursing practice here can be problematic. Course content, such as health assessment, pathophysiology, leadership, and research, may be universal, but content for nursing care-related courses, health policy, clinical courses, and even skills-related courses may require a strong foundation that is based on nursing practice in the United States. International faculty may need support in speaking and writing in the English language. Resources to assist in these areas should be mobilized early to promote success in the faculty role.

Gauging the content expertise of any new faculty member is important. That person may have expertise that does not necessarily "fit" with courses that are currently "open." Faculty members should not have a sense of ownership for the specific courses they are teaching. Academic leaders and faculty alike cannot take the position that new faculty will simply "fill in" current holes in the teaching schedule. When new faculty are hired, they may have credentials that outweigh those faculty currently teaching certain courses. For example, a new faculty member who previously practiced as an adult-gerontology nurse practitioner or one who is certified in geriatric nursing may be a better option to teach a geriatrics course than a faculty member whose nursing career involved working for some years in a long-term care setting. Faculty who have more recent clinical experience in a specialty may be more suited to teach a specialty course than one whose clinical experiences are more remote. Faculty who have a research agenda that aligns with a course or courses would be expected to teach students in those areas. Advanced degrees, certifications, research experience, or other credentials to identify and support expertise in certain areas are important criteria for accreditation and justifying how faculty teaching loads are determined.

Just as in healthcare, cross-training is good so that when new faculty are brought in, current faculty understand they may have to alter their teaching loads to accommodate the expertise of new faculty. Some schools have policies in place that a faculty member will be allowed to teach a course two to three times when first assigned. After that, the course becomes fair game for someone else who may have preferred credentials or who may have a passion for the topic, if credentials are not a determinant for a teaching assignment. Having a policy that allows a person to teach a course for at least two to three offerings ensures that a person can prep for a course, teach it, evaluate it, and then make necessary revisions. As an academic leader, one should establish such policies or practices early before they may need to be enacted. Change can be difficult for some faculty members, especially if a new faculty member is assigned to teaching "their course." In most SON, it is expected that course materials will be shared with a new faculty member assigned to teach a course.

Having a diverse faculty and staff can only enrich the SON and contribute to a culture of inclusivity. Taylor et al. (2010) lists recommendations for recruiting and retaining diverse faculty. These are listed in Box 5.5.

Box 5.5 Recommendations for Diversifying Faculty

- One strategy will not work at all institutions
- Institutions must match what they say about diversity and their actions related to diversity
- Student diversity enhances faculty diversity
- Policies, procedures, and processes related to diversity should be explicit

(continued)

Box 5.5 Recommendations for Diversifying Faculty (*continued*)

- A curriculum and research priorities that focus on diversity can attract diverse faculty
- The campus, departmental, and community culture must reflect a commitment to diversity
- Recruitment strategies for diverse faculty have to be followed by strong mentorship and support for advancement within the university when diverse faculty are hired

The strategies listed here can be applied to staff as well. Understanding the breadth and depth that comes from thinking differently and challenging each other to expand our thoughts and our minds is enhanced when those from diverse backgrounds come together to enrich the lives of students in their educational endeavors. Although private schools will ensure all faculty fit the mission of the organization, this should not preclude hiring diverse faculty and staff.

REFERENCES

Brown, S. (2016, October 28). Tenure denials among minority faculty members set off alarms, and a book, about obstacles for minority faculty. *Chronicle of Higher Education*, p. A8.

Finkelstein, M., Conley, V., & Schuster, J. (2016, April). Taking the measure of faculty diversity. *Advancing Higher Education*. New York, NY: Teachers Insurance and Annuity Association of America Institute.

Flaherty, C. (2016, August 22). More faculty diversity, not on tenure track. Retrieved from https://www.insidehighered.com/news/2016/08/22/study-finds-gains-faculty-diversity-not-tenure-track

Goldrick-Rab, S. (2016, May 20). What does a genuine commitment to diversity look like? *Chronicle of Higher Education*, p. A25.

Harper, S. R. (2016, May 20). What does a genuine commitment to diversity look like? *Chronicle of Higher Education*, p. A25.

Lynch, M. (2013, April 24). Diversity in college faculty just as important as student body. *Diverse Issues in Higher Education*. Retrieved from http://diverseeducation.com/article/52902

McMurtrie, B. (2016, September 16). How to do a better job of searching for diversity. *Chronicle of Higher Education*, pp. A20–A25.

Pink, D. (2011). *Drive: The surprising truth about what motivates us*. New York, NY: Riverhead Books.

Schmidt, P. (2016, May 20). Demand surges for diversity consultants. *Chronicle of Higher Education*, pp. A14–A15.

Smith, D. (2009). Reframing diversity as an institutional capacity. *Diversity and Democracy*, 12(2). Retrieved from https://www.aacu.org/publications -research/periodicals/reframing-diversity-institutional-capacity

Snyder, T. D., de Brey, C., & Dillow, S. A. (2016). *Digest of education statistics, 2015 (NCES 2016-014, 51st ed.)*. Washington, DC: National Center for Education Statistics, Institute of Education Sciences, U.S. Department of Education.

Taylor, O., Burgan Apprey, C., Hill, G., McGrann, L., & Wang, J. (2010). Diversifying the faculty. *peerReview, 12*(3). Retrieved from https://www .aacu.org/publications-research/periodicals/diversifying-faculty

Trower, C. (2010). A new generation of faculty: Similar core values in a different world. *peerReview, 12*(3). Retrieved from https://www.aacu .org/publications-research/periodicals/new-generation-faculty-similar -core-values-different-world

Wilde, J., & Finkelstein, J. (2016, November 25). Hiring a search firm? Do your homework first. *Chronicle of Higher Education*, p. A25.

CHAPTER 6

MARKETING AND PUBLIC RELATIONS

All schools have to rely on marketing and public relations to publicize their accomplishments and to attract students, faculty, and staff. The trend today is to "brand" organizations so that the public can readily identify them and associate the brand with something they remember about the organization. Chapter 4 discussed how nursing faculty and administrators are involved in attracting donors and alumni. This chapter focuses more on general audiences but there is some overlap between how schools and universities market to potential donors and to potential students and employees.

■ THE PUBLIC UNIVERSITY PERSPECTIVE

The public university school of nursing (SON) must always consider the budget implications of marketing and public relations. The SON may choose to reserve some money to pay for printing or to buy give-away items. The amount will depend on how much responsibility the SON has for marketing and advertising the SON. Public relations typically fall within the marketing department, which can be very busy and understaffed, particularly in a large public university. However, learn the university and system policies regarding how the unit or SON is expected to utilize the marketing department.

Consequently, the SON may be expected and encouraged to engage in some minor marketing activities. The marketing department might even have a self-help option that the SON can access online. This might be used to develop brochures or business cards. However, the university, particularly the chancellor or president, is responsible for establishing what the university branding will be and what the university's tagline or key message should be. My author colleague, Dr. Chappy, discusses branding in more detail later in this chapter. However, once the "brand" is determined, the SON and other units must be consistent with that brand. So, everyone must use the same branded letterhead and the same university logo, and so forth.

Just as the university must explore what makes it unique so it can accurately and effectively sell its brand, the SON should also identify what makes it unique or special. For many years, SON used a particular nursing theory or conceptual framework to support the mission and vision. Most SON have moved away from that but it is still necessary, perhaps now more than ever when there is so much more competition among schools, to define what is special about the SON. Is community engagement particularly important? Maybe it is interprofessional education, work with vulnerable populations, or innovation. It can be almost anything but the SON must be able to put their money where its mouth is. That is, if the SON claims to be focused on community engagement, then it should be clear to the public that students and faculty have a variety of opportunities to engage with the community in unique and innovative ways.

Determining what is special about the SON is challenging because practically all accredited SON strive to provide an excellent education to students, for high NCLEX® and certification pass rates, for inclusivity and diversity and to be innovative. Although high board pass rates are laudable, the public does not understand how critical it is to have a high pass rate. The public may not even be aware that it should be considering the SON's NCLEX and certification pass rates when evaluating an SON. The public, including potential students and their parents, assume that the SON will educate the student to become a practicing nurse. Experienced RNs seeking graduate education may be only slightly more informed about how to evaluate the quality of an SON. We often forget that the public does not "speak" nursing and doesn't really know how to distinguish among nursing programs. The public does not understand why nursing has multiple points of entry into the profession or what all of the letters after our names signify. We often don't know ourselves! Try to view your websites and other public information through the public's eyes and make it very clear why your SON is the best choice.

The SON should have a good working relationship with the university marketing department. This author found that monthly meetings to discuss events happening in the SON enabled the marketing professionals to determine what should be publicized and by what means. While dean at one SON, I led preparations for a grand opening of a new building, including the dedication of a history wall and installation of a time capsule, a 50th anniversary of the SON, and the annual nursing fund-raising event. The advancement or development officer (see Chapter 4) and faculty/staff committees were extremely helpful in these efforts, but it was the marketing department on whom we relied to design the "save the date" cards, publicize the event, and develop the event program brochures. Professional-looking marketing materials can make all of the difference.

Many legislators and regents visited the SON because of our grand opening and our cutting-edge facilities and simulators. Again, these groups do not typically have much knowledge of nursing beyond understanding that there is always a nursing shortage and that their constituents need more nurses to care for them. The message you convey to them should be succinct, clear, and consistent. Faculty, staff, and students who join the chief nurse executive to give tours or greet distinguished guests should be trained to help deliver the message.

This author's message was always consistent: The citizens of this state (and across the nation) are aging, nurses and nurse educators are preparing to retire, there are not enough doctorally prepared nurses to educate new nurses, and there will not be enough RNs to care for the citizens of the state. The simulation technician and the simulation educator were advised to give brief explanations of how the simulators worked and how they added to student learning. They needed reminders that this particular audience wanted to hear that the money they lobbied for to renovate or build a new facility was well spent and that the new facility and the equipment were significantly impacting nursing education. The ability to tailor what was said about the simulators, depending on the audience, became a valuable skill given the short amount of time designated to these tours and visits.

One of this author's goals when assuming this particular dean role was to increase the visibility of the SON. In addition to working with marketing and the information technology specialist to revamp the website to be more navigable, we added "points of pride" on the opening page of the website. We continued to add to this as our accomplishments accumulated. We posted short video clips and stories of faculty and students to highlight their work and innovative activities. Later in this chapter, Dr. Chappy writes in more detail about using websites for marketing.

Another way to increase visibility is to have faculty bring fliers to conferences. Large standing banners and small table-top banners that display the SON brand and the types of programs it offers are also effective. These can be carried to conferences. The younger generation of students generally prefers the Internet to paper. Business-type cards with the SON website printed on them are an attractive option. Students tend to love pens, sometimes in the shape of a syringe, notepads, and other small items that bear the SON logo. You may find it helpful to survey students formally or informally to find out what kinds of items they think prospective students would prefer. Your student nurses' association can provide helpful feedback.

The SON may already have an annual publication that is geared primarily to alumni and donors, but is also often made available to other SON in the region or across the country. This newsletter or magazine highlights the accomplishments and interesting stories from the past year. It typically includes a section on faculty publications and presentations. The purpose of the magazine or newsletter is to demonstrate that the SON is fulfilling its mission and accomplishing great things.

Another idea that this author found very useful is the quarterly electronic newsletter sent to all involved with the university, its alumni, and donors. I included a dean's message that allowed me to highlight SON accomplishments, recognize specific people for their work, and announce new initiatives. Because it was electronic, we were able to link to stories on the website to encourage readers to learn more. It was particularly gratifying to highlight stories of student success and innovation.

Social media is another tool used by SON to reach students, in particular. Most SON have a social media policy and although it is targeted to students, faculty and staff should also observe the social media policy. Appointing one person with an interest in social media who is knowledgeable about social media to coordinate these efforts, collect the stories and announcements, and post them is the key to success. This person should also vet announcements, stories, and pictures from others to ensure that the SON continues to convey a professional image.

The Press

A savvy nurse administrator takes advantage of every opportunity to increase the visibility of the SON. New programs, services, technology, and personnel, among other things, may be items of interest to print or post using other media. This is one reason to have regular meetings with the university marketing department. This department can help you sort out what would be of interest and it can contact the appropriate news outlet.

This author was surprised on more than one occasion by a call or email from university marketing to say that a reporter would appear in the office within the hour and to be prepared to be on camera. This always seemed to happen on the rare occasions I dressed casually for work.

I learned to keep some extra makeup and a scarf in my office, just in case. Apparently, it is discovered that there is time to fill for the evening news so the reporter does the story with little advance notice to the interviewee. Having brief talking points, such as those mentioned earlier, can be helpful in a pinch. More than likely, the press is coming to see you because of something new and newsworthy. In any case, if it is something newsworthy about the SON, you will probably know much more about it than the television news can fit into the time slot. As you prepare, focus on what you really think the public should know about the event. Why is it newsworthy? Try to slip in some words about how the event/program will enhance nursing education or the nursing profession and why it makes your SON stand out from all the others. Exploit the opportunity as much as possible to highlight why your SON and this particular event/program is the best.

Radio interviews present their own challenges. In this author's experience, there is usually sufficient (2 or 3 days) notice to prepare answers to predetermined interview questions; however, the radio spot is typically live so editing is not an option. The interviewer may also add or change questions based on the course of your dialogue and in response to callers. Remember that you know the subject better than the audience or you would not be the person being interviewed. Keep answers brief and concise and wait for the interviewer to probe a topic further if he or she feels it needs elaboration. In this author's experience, one is given a time, date, and a number to call. On calling the phone number, you will be able to hear the disc jockey or radio announcer speaking to the audience or you might hear a commercial. The announcer may or may not speak to you before you go live. In my case, the interviews were live as soon as the radio announcer started speaking to me. Try to just focus on speaking with the announcer. These are typically very experienced people who know what audiences want to hear about and how to make you comfortable.

Newspaper and other print media interviews tend to be less rushed. It is helpful to know a little about the perspective and the typical audience of the newspaper. If you are unfamiliar, ask the reporter/journalist some questions that will enlighten you about how the paper tends to view nurses and healthcare providers. If you have time, peruse articles online. Nobody does not like nurses so the topic of nursing is unlikely to be controversial. However, whether or not to implement healthcare reforms and how, and the high costs and expectations of insurance companies and big pharma are controversial. Depending on the topic on which you are being interviewed, you may be asked to comment, so think about the current healthcare issues of the day and decide how you would respond if asked. It is not unreasonable to expect that you might be asked to comment on controversial healthcare issues or trends even if these are not pertinent to the original topic of discussion. Whatever the issue about which you are interviewed, take the opportunity to talk about your SON and why it is special. Try to add how nursing relates to the future of healthcare and why resources, such as grants, are needed to continue to fund nursing education.

Do not hesitate to correct misconceptions if you encounter them during TV, radio, or print press interviews. During one radio interview, the radio announcer made an erroneous comment about the nursing profession. This author corrected the announcer before answering the next question. Although interviewing for television, print media, or radio is unnerving, these are excellent opportunities to increase the visibility of your SON and to speak on behalf of nursing. The public is still exposed to misleading images of nursing. Although the public image of nursing has significantly improved, it is not always based on reality. Remember the popular television daytime show during which a celebrity asked why a beauty contestant who is a nurse was wearing a stethoscope? Nurses everywhere rallied to show off their stethoscopes. Opportunities to speak for nursing and nursing education come up in the most unexpected and unusual ways.

■ THE FOR-PROFIT UNIVERSITY PERSPECTIVE

Marketing is a priority in the for-profit sector because success is evaluated at least in part by the relationship between operating expenses and income, which is generated by enrollment. No enrollment, no income. For-profits generally open schools in areas where there is a known market demand. However, the market needs to know you are there and what you have to offer. Once established, word of mouth will help grow the program and in most cases new start-ups have more applicants than capacity, but in order to sustain that level of interest and expand, you have to create a compelling case for choosing your program over your competitors. The for-profits have some real challenges as they tend to be more expensive and have shorter track records with the boards of nursing. A carefully constructed and robust marketing campaign is essential to success and therefore best managed by the marketing department. This is especially true in the for-profit sector as for-profit schools are highly scrutinized by the Federal Trade Commission (FTC) to be sure they are in compliance with Section 5 of the FTC Act, which prohibits unfair or deceptive practices affecting commerce. In 2013, the FTC revised their guidelines related to private vocational and distance education programs and their advertising practices. Selected revised guidelines for Section 5 provided in 16 CFR (Code of Federal Regulations) part 254 of the *Federal Register* are presented in Table 6.1.

Table 6.1 Selected Revised Guidelines Pertaining to Private Vocational and Distance Education Programs

Section	Current Language
254.1 Definitions	(a) Accredited. A school or program of instruction that has been evaluated and found to meet established criteria by an accrediting agency or association recognized for such purposes by the U.S. Department of Education. (b) Approved. A school or program of instruction that has been recognized by a State or Federal agency as meeting educational standards or other related qualifications as prescribed by that agency for the school or program of instruction to which the term is applied. The term is not and should not be used interchangeably with "Accredited." The term "Approved" is not justified by the mere grant of a corporate charter to operate or license to do business as a school and should not be used unless the represented "approval" has been affirmatively required or authorized by State or Federal law. (c) Industry member. Industry Members are the persons, firms, corporations, or organizations covered by these Guides, as explained in §254.0(a)
254.3 Misrepresentation of Extent or Nature of Accreditation or Approval	(a) It is deceptive for an Industry Member to misrepresent, directly or indirectly, expressly or by implication, the nature, extent, or purpose of any Approval by a State or Federal agency or Accreditation by an accrediting agency or association. For example, an Industry Member should not: (1) Represent, without qualification, that its school is Accredited unless all courses and programs of instruction have been Accredited by an accrediting agency recognized by the U.S. Department of Education. If an Accredited school offers courses or programs of instruction that are not Accredited, all advertisements or promotional materials pertaining to those courses or programs, and making reference to the Accreditation of the school, should clearly and conspicuously disclose that those particular courses or programs are not Accredited.

(continued)

Table 6.1   Selected Revised Guidelines Pertaining to Private Vocational and Distance Education Programs (*continued*)

Section	Current Language
	(2) Represent that its school or program of instruction is Approved, unless the nature, extent, and purpose of that Approval are disclosed. (3) Misrepresent the extent to which a student successfully completing a course or program of instruction will be able to transfer any credits the student earns to any other postsecondary institution. (b) It is deceptive for an Industry Member to misrepresent, directly or indirectly, expressly or by implication, that a school or program of instruction has been Approved by a particular industry, or that successful completion of a course or program of instruction qualifies the student for admission to a labor union or similar organization or for receiving a State or Federal license to perform certain functions. (c) It is deceptive for an Industry Member to misrepresent, directly or indirectly, expressly or by implication, that its courses or programs of instruction are recommended by vocational counselors, high schools, colleges, educational organizations, employment agencies, or members of a particular industry, or that it has been the subject of unsolicited testimonials or endorsements from former students. It is deceptive for an Industry Member to use testimonials or endorsements that do not accurately reflect current practices of the school or current conditions or employment opportunities in the industry or occupation for which students are being trained. Note to paragraph (c): The Commission's Guides Concerning Use of Endorsements and Testimonials in Advertising (part 255 of this chapter) provide further guidance in this area. (d) It is deceptive for an Industry Member to misrepresent, directly or indirectly, expressly or by implication, that its courses or programs of instruction fulfill a requirement that must be completed prior to taking a licensing examination.

Section	Current Language
254.4 Misrepresentation of Facilities	Misrepresentation of facilities, services, qualifications of staff, status, and employment prospects for students after training. (a) It is deceptive for an Industry Member to misrepresent, directly or indirectly, expressly or by implication, in advertising, promotional materials, recruitment sessions, or in any other manner, the size, location, services, facilities, curriculum, books and materials, or equipment of its school or the number or educational qualifications of its faculty and other personnel. For example, an Industry Member should not: (1) Misrepresent the qualifications, credentials, experience, or educational background of its instructors, sales representatives, or other employees. (2) Misrepresent, through statements or pictures, or in any other manner, the nature or efficacy of its courses, training devices, methods, or equipment. (3) Misrepresent the availability of employment while the student is undergoing instruction or the role of the school in providing or arranging for such employment. (4) Misrepresent the availability, amount, or nature of any financial assistance available to students, including any Federal student financial assistance. If the cost of training is financed in whole or in part by loans, students should be informed that loans must be repaid whether or not they are successful in completing the program and obtaining employment. (5) Misrepresent that a private entity providing any financial assistance to the students is part of the Federal government or that loans from the private entity have the same interest rate or repayment terms as loans received from the U.S. Department of Education. (6) Misrepresent the nature of any relationship between the school or its personnel and any government agency, or that students of the school will receive preferred consideration for employment with any government agency.

(*continued*)

Table 6.1   Selected Revised Guidelines Pertaining to Private Vocational and Distance Education Programs (*continued*)

Section	Current Language
	(7) Misrepresent that certain individuals or classes of individuals are members of its faculty or advisory board, have prepared instructional materials, or are otherwise affiliated with the school. (8) Misrepresent the nature and extent of any personal instruction, guidance, assistance, or other service, including placement assistance and assistance overcoming language barriers or learning disabilities, it will provide students either during or after completion of a course. (9) Misrepresent the extent to which a prospective student will receive credit for courses or a program of instruction already completed at other postsecondary institutions. (10) Misrepresent the percentage of students who withdraw from a course or program of instruction, or the percentage of students who complete or graduate from a course or program of instruction. (11) Misrepresent security policies or crime statistics that the school must maintain. (b) It is deceptive for an Industry Member to misrepresent, directly or indirectly, expressly or by implication, that it is a nonprofit organization or that it is affiliated or otherwise connected with any public institution or private religious or charitable organization. (c) It is deceptive for an Industry Member that conducts its instruction by correspondence, or other form of distance education, to fail to clearly and conspicuously disclose that fact in all promotional materials. (d) It is deceptive for an Industry Member to misrepresent, directly or indirectly, expressly or by implication, that a course or program of instruction has been recently revised or instructional equipment is up-to-date, or misrepresent its ability to keep a course or program of instruction current and up-to-date.

Section	Current Language
	(e) It is deceptive for an Industry Member, in promoting any course or program of instruction in its advertising, promotional materials, or in any other manner, to misrepresent, directly or indirectly, expressly or by implication, whether through the use of text, images, endorsements, or by other means, the availability of employment after graduation from a school or program of instruction, the specific type of employment available to a student after graduation from a school or program of instruction, the success that the Industry Member's graduates have realized in obtaining such employment, including the percentage of graduates who have received employment, or the salary or salary range that the Industry Member's graduates have received, or can be expected to receive, in such employment. Note to paragraph (e): The Commission's Guides Concerning Use of Endorsements and Testimonials in Advertising (part 255 of this chapter) provide further guidance in this area.
§ 254.7 Deceptive Sales Practices	(a) It is deceptive for an Industry Member to use advertisements or promotional materials that misrepresent, directly or indirectly, expressly or by implication, that employment is being offered or that a talent hunt or contest is being conducted. For example, captions such as, "Men/women wanted to train for * * * ," "Help Wanted," "Employment," "Business Opportunities," and words or terms of similar import, may falsely convey that employment is being offered and therefore should be avoided.(b) It is deceptive for an Industry Member to fail to disclose to a prospective student, before enrollment, the total cost of the program of instruction and the school's refund policy if the student does not complete the program of instruction.(c) It is deceptive for an Industry Member to fail to disclose to a prospective student, prior to enrollment, all requirements for successfully completing the course or program of instruction and the circumstances that would constitute grounds for terminating the student's enrollment prior to completion of the program of instruction.

These guidelines require strict adherence. Making any claim that cannot be substantiated with the purpose of enticing students can and does result in hefty fines and in some cases repayment of tuition and forgiveness of loans (Douglas-Gabriel, 2016). These claims can be as simple as stating that your program is the largest in the nation or that you have the best placement rate. In addition, in schools that are publicly traded any disclosure that could affect the success of the program could affect its value in the stock market and therefore could violate Securities and Exchange Commission (SEC) rules. Therefore, all public communications should originate or be vetted by the marketing and public relations department(s).

Marketing is messaging and involves not only what to communicate, but how, where, to whom, and how often to communicate. No matter how well written, an ad will not be effective if it does not reach its target audience. Figuring out who that audience is today is much more challenging than it used to be. Students choosing to attend for-profit schools belong to all age groups, ethnicities, and military statuses, and include persons who are digital natives and digital immigrants. For some groups the medium is not just the way to deliver a message it *is* the message. Sending "tweets" via Twitter, for example, sends a message that you can relate to and meet the needs of a certain demographic just by using that means of communication. Of course, only those with Twitter accounts will receive the message. Most for-profits have a team that focuses solely on managing social media both in terms of marketing and image management. Program leaders receive regular feedback about what is being shared in social media about the program and are expected to follow up with current students who are found making negative comments about the school or posting items or statements that are inconsistent with the school's code of conduct. A rule of thumb is that it takes 10 positive comments to counteract a single negative one. For-profit programs are less well known than larger universities and therefore creating positive "buzz" in social media will help increase the applicant pool. In addition, the for-profits generally pay search engines to be among the first schools that appear when potential applicants search for a SON.

In terms of public relations, for-profits are continually battling "negative press" and seek to counteract that by highlighting student success stories and community service. Like their counterparts, for-profits generally have a department that interacts with any outside individual or company requesting information about our programs or our graduates. This department is also continually on the lookout for stories to pitch to the media like campus anniversaries, legislative days, student involvement in charities, and so on. Campus leaders are wise to look ahead for things that the media will likely be covering anyway, such as National Women's History Month, Earth Day, and Heart Month, and plan along with the public relations team to do something to get media attention.

The way in which students, and equally important (if not more so) the clinical faculty, are perceived by the staff nurses and unit managers can make or break your reputation in the healthcare community. Leadership needs to visit clinical sites, engage practice partners by including them on their advisory boards or regular meetings designed to share common concerns. That faculty and leadership should respond quickly to any student issues from parking to appearance to actual practice concerns. If there are local consortiums, area-wide dean's meetings, Internet collaboratives, and so on, attend those and make use of any opportunity to collaborate on pilot projects, research, and health fairs. Another opportunity to enhance the brand is by participating on professional committees at the national, state, and local levels.

■ THE PRIVATE UNIVERSITY PERSPECTIVE

Marketing and public relations are different facets used for advertising university and school programs and services so others will gain interest in the university, school, and their offerings with the hopes that they will become consumers or even benefactors. Marketing and public relations efforts are critical in getting a clear, correct, and consistent message to internal and external stakeholders about the university, the school, programs, curricular offerings, and cocurricular activities. Aspects related to student life in the marketing message may contribute to choosing which school to attend, as are the majors and minors offered. Marketing and public relations seek to attract potential students, and in the case of undergraduate students, convince their parents and families that spending the additional money that it costs to attend a private school are well worth the investment.

Marketing efforts should have a well-recognized brand, something that distinguishes the university from its competitors. A brand can include a logo or emblem that viewers will associate with the school. This creates recognizability and conveys a positive image. We all can think of brands for athletic wear, airlines, and other goods and services that we regularly use in our everyday lives that we immediately recognize and can name the company that manufactures those items or provides the services. We can also name brands for goods and services that we may have never used because the companies that manufacture them do an excellent job of getting a well-recognized and well-defined brand in their advertising initiatives. For private schools, their brand should be associated with their mission, and should convey a positive image to connect viewers with the university. Some schools will work directly with marketing specialists to craft a well-perceived brand that will then be evident in all marketing materials.

At this author's university, there was a merger of two campuses in 2013. These two separate universities, which were part of the same system, were coming together as one university with two residential campuses. It was critical to create a new brand that encompassed both campuses, whereas at the same time not losing the individualized uniqueness that each campus offered. Much time and effort was spent on this, with great attention paid to not losing the market and followers who were already familiar with the "old" brands of each individual campus.

Typically, a certain percentage of the operating budget or a certain dollar amount per year is dedicated to marketing. Nursing leaders need to decide how to allocate those dollars to get the most value. At this author's university, approximately 2% of the annual budget is allocated toward marketing and public relations. Although many individuals or groups may be targeted by marketing materials, critically important stakeholders are current and potential students (and their families, in many cases), current and potential faculty and staff, and other users of university services. Marketing materials are, by design, intended to showcase the school and what it has to offer in the hopes that it will draw more users to the school. Users can include not only those potential traditional undergraduate and graduate students, but also parents and families of potential students. Others include nontraditional users of university or school services such as those who will pursue certificate or other educational programs, those who will attend university concerts, sporting events, or plays, as well as potential employers of the students or the school's graduates.

As for effective marketing, all private schools tend to tout smaller class sizes and more personalized and individualized attention to students. Faith-based schools tend to include connections with a religious affiliation. So private schools have to ensure they are creating marketing materials that emphasize what makes them unique, not only from other private schools, but also from their much cheaper public university counterparts. Using the mission as a central theme, private school leaders can develop marketing materials that will show their unique niche in the educational market. That said, private schools want to develop marketing materials to appeal to the widest possible audience. We value diversity of thought; however, all students are exposed to the mission and principles underpinning the mission, not in an effort to convert students, but in an effort to be mission-minded. On a recent end-of-program survey, one student commented that he or she thought there was too much emphasis on religion. That comment made me wonder why the student chose our university for his or her education, but at the same time, it supported that faculty and staff were indeed living the university's mission by emphasizing religiosity in every class.

There are many reasons why potential students tend to enroll in programs and other offerings at private universities. These can include the university's geographic location, the reputation of its graduates, specific programs and curricular offerings (majors, minors, and certificates), its admission and progression policies, or its cocurricular activities like sports programs or study-abroad options that may not be available at competing universities. A good marketing plan will capitalize on all of these aspects in various marketing endeavors or when marketing to various audiences. Students who have a passion for athletics or theater and who may not have the abilities or talent to participate in such activities at a large public university may excel in a smaller private university (little fish in a big pond vs. big fish in a little pond). Some student athletes will forgo opportunities to be a reserve on a team at a large school in exchange for attending a smaller private school in which they will be able to have a career as a starter, or even be a star on a team. Some very academically gifted students may not be socially comfortable in a large public university setting and may choose to attend a smaller private university. Some students choose a private university because they sense a strong connection with the mission.

Certainly, marketing materials for different programs must convey a unique message that will attract those audiences who may be most interested in attending that program. Marketing an undergraduate program must have different strategies than marketing a graduate or certificate program. Marketing that targets high school students and their parents is very different than marketing to target adult learners or career changers. So again, marketing niche services must be directed to the widest potential audiences but must be specifically relevant to those with the greatest potential to become students or users of the services that the university offers.

Academic leaders must remember that educational institutions are all competing for the same students. Changes in demographics of the regional population (decreased numbers of high school students) or in the economy (higher or lower unemployment rates) can trigger even fiercer competition. At this author's institution, in an effort to ramp up marketing to potential traditional undergraduate students who may have a strong connection to the mission, our university initiated a campaign specifically directed toward those potential undergraduate students who are members of a particular religious congregation.

When marketing, leaders should ask: What is the best way to reach the target audience? For example, potential students for a bachelor of science in nursing (BSN) completion program would most likely be associate-degree-prepared nurses working within healthcare systems or those currently enrolled in an associate degree or diploma nursing program. Potential master's degree students would be those who are currently enrolled in a bachelor's degree program or those who are currently working within a healthcare system or agency as a bachelor's-prepared registered nurse. Those potential students for a doctoral program would be those nurses who are currently master's prepared or, in the case of BSN-to-DNP (doctor of nursing practice) or BSN-to-PhD programs, would be current students in a baccalaureate program or bachelor's-prepared registered nurses looking to advance within the nursing profession. It could be effective to market BSN completion or graduate programs at a National Student Nurses Association meeting, in which attendees are enrolled in either associate degree or bachelor's degree programs, but it would not be wise to market a traditional undergraduate program at such a conference. Similarly, advertising a doctoral program at a master's education conference makes sense. Scholarly conferences, such as those sponsored by Sigma Theta Tau International or a regional nursing research society, would have attendees most likely more interested in graduate education (master's or doctoral) but not those interested in a baccalaureate program. So, when spending marketing dollars, it is critical to ensure that the intended message is getting to the correctly intended audience.

Many healthcare organizations strive to hire more baccalaureate-prepared nurses if they are seeking Magnet® status or are attempting to meet the Institute of Medicine's recommendation for an 80% BSN-prepared workforce. Thus, advertising BSN completion programs within healthcare organizations can show benefits. With working nurses, marketing materials should reflect how completing the BSN degree at a particular school can fit into an already busy lifestyle. Showcasing why your program may be more flexible or can be completed in a shorter period of time may be beneficial. Sometimes marketing efforts may be held in check until after a significant curriculum revision or other innovations that could set a program apart from others in the area that are competitors. That way, dollars may be better spent to tout the updates or innovations.

Websites are key venues from which potential students and other stakeholders get information about the school and its programs. Having an up-to-date website that is easy to navigate shares information with internal and external stakeholders. Using consultants and marketing personnel with specific expertise related to website development and maintenance ensures that users can access the types of information they seek. Some websites have too much information; others have too little. Finding the correct balance is key for an effective website that does not look too cluttered or too barren. Websites must be continually maintained and updated along with ensuring that "old" information gets deleted and will not "show up" when users are searching for a particular item. Therefore, SON often need a person within the department with the knowledge and skills to add content to a website or to delete old content to keep it current. Website analytics help determine what information is being accessed by visitors to the site, what information is not being accessed, how much time people are spending on various components within the website, and other key information regarding the website usage. Using such data to drive decisions about website revision and maintenance will help to justify marketing-budget adjustments.

Digital marketing has become a significantly more cost-effective and efficient investment with the potential to reach a much wider audience as compared to using print media. One reason that digital marketing is appealing is that changes can be made easily to reflect program updates or changes. If a school is using brochures to market its programs, even a small change to a program could necessitate reprinting several hundred brochures. Often schools will update brochures annually, and this may not be soon enough to convey changes to intended users. The last thing academic leaders want is to have inaccurate information getting to intended students.

Sometimes very simple and no-cost investments of time can make a difference in marketing a program or trying to convey a message to potential users. For example, a phone call from a faculty member or dean to those who have applied to the nursing program but have not yet committed to the university or are undecided about their school selection can create a strong connection that could sway the student to enroll in the school. One student admitted that he was highly sought by several universities, but when a faculty member personally called him and encouraged him to select this caller's school, that was the deciding factor. Sometimes student workers can be used to call applicants and they are very eager and capable of telling applicants about the student experience at the school and why attending there is the right choice. This student-to-potential-student contact can be very compelling when applicants are deciding where to enroll. Of course, it is best to use some sort of script or phone call template when using student workers to ensure the message that is delivered is the intended message and the message is consistent. Student workers can always direct unanswered question to the dean or to a faculty member, which could lead to an additional point of contact.

Academic leaders can expect to work closely with the marketing team. The marketing team has the skills and abilities to "get the message out" in an appealing manner, but they need input and assistance from academic leaders to ensure that facts, figures, and the overall message about the academic program are correct. The marketing team will not have expertise in nursing, academic programming, or even who the intended audience should be, so academic leaders and the marketing team need a close working relationship. There should be a mutual respect and understanding to critique and correct each other's ideas and work products so that the information conveyed in marketing materials is appealing, meaningful, accurate, and getting out to the intended audience.

Sometimes working with the marketing team involves give-and-take whereby budget dollars originally intended for the SON need to be reallocated throughout the university. The SON and other schools may not have their own individual marketing budgets. Sometimes priorities need to be made in which those in the SON will give up a share of their budget to support marketing new or updated programs from another department or division. Potential returns on investment should always be considered in such deliberations, and it should be made known that SON priorities will need attention again in the future. Marketing has to be ongoing, or schools and programs will see dips in enrollment due to lack of visibility.

Using social media for marketing has been addressed earlier in this chapter. However, one facet that was not addressed was using things like Facebook Live to broadcast live events. A grand opening, a service project, a student's presentation or other events could be streamed to those who may wish to attend but physically cannot be at the event in person. Live streaming a grand-opening event or other campus activities can engage people using social media to showcase an event at little to no cost.

Public relations can take many forms. Universities and their student bodies are "neighbors" within a community. How the community accepts the university and its students can vary. Sometimes, especially if a university and its student population grows, there can be challenges with being a "good neighbor" and living in peace with the surrounding community. For example, growth of a university may mean adding an athletic field, and lights for that athletic field could be disruptive to neighbors. Therefore, involving neighbors in planning and development of aspects related to student life and university strategic planning that can impact neighbors is critical to the success of existing and new or proposed initiatives. It can often be easier to get along with neighbors who move into the area after the school and its facilities are established rather than having neighbors who are established and then adding new facilities that could affect the status quo. Neighbors might be upset if they suddenly or over time face increased traffic, more litter around their properties, more noise from student activities or other things that are disruptive to what the neighbors were used to. Therefore, any type of outreach and getting the neighbors involved and on board with university activities is time well spent.

Sometimes public relations means working to mend a damaged reputation. An incident at the school or even an incident with one single student can lead to negative reactions among neighbors, community partners, clinical partners, and others who interact with the school and its students. When this author began her current role as dean, one particular clinic refused to take our nurse practitioner (NP) students for clinical rotations because of a past incident involving pretty significant issues. I worked very hard to meet with leaders at that clinic to investigate what happened, and to ensure that the problems that led to the incidents had been rectified. In addition, I highlighted recent curricular revisions that would make our student outcomes even better. Although the clinic now takes our students in NP rotations, it took effort and open communication to mend the damaged relationship. Of course, we want to convey a positive and successful image to all of our clinical partners, but when a bad experience occurred in the past, relationships need to be nurtured in an even stronger manner. That is the only way to win back or restore trust.

Public relations may also include advocating for initiatives through writing to or meeting with legislators regarding policy proposals that could affect the school or its students. Academic leaders should be clear in meetings or letters if they are representing the school or representing themselves during encounters with elected officials. It is best to represent the school, because even if academic leaders say that they are representing themselves, they will be associated with the school. In a private school, leaders have to be careful that political stances, when conveyed publicly, are not contradictory to the school's mission, again realizing that mission is at the center of everything, including actions outside of work.

As noted in other chapters, it is often the dean of the SON who is seen as the face of the school. Therefore, every appearance, all actions, and words spoken in public can be seen as public relations events. Academic leaders have to be sure that behaviors, words, and actions are consistent with the mission and congruent with a positive marketing or public relations message.

REFERENCE

Douglas-Gabriel, D. (2016, December 15). DeVry agrees to $100 million settlement with the FTC. *Washington Post*. Retrieved from https:// www.washingtonpost.com/news/grade-point/wp/2016/12/15/devry -agrees-to-100-million-settlement-with-the-ftc/?utm_term=.377cf14909a3

CHAPTER 7

DEVELOPING AND SUSTAINING CLINICAL PARTNERSHIPS AND FACULTY PRACTICE

Clinical partnerships are vital to the success of any nursing program. Students must have sites in which to learn real-life nursing with human patients. Simulated experiences are excellent to help students learn new skills and begin to develop safe practice; however, there is no substitute for working with real patients and with other members of the healthcare team.

Similarly, faculty frequently want to maintain their own clinical skills and may want to engage in some form of faculty practice. Other schools of nursing (SON) may require faculty practice. SON define *application* (Boyer, 1990) differently, so might have no requirement or vague guidelines.

■ THE PUBLIC UNIVERSITY PERSPECTIVE

Faculty and academic nurse leaders play significant roles in developing, strengthening, and sustaining clinical partnerships. They are ambassadors for the SON and frequently engage in their own clinical practice ("faculty practice") in partner organizations. Clinical partnerships are vital to the success of an SON. Developing and cultivating these partnerships must be high priorities (Box 7.1).

Many schools across the country are now being asked to pay for these clinical placements. This has occurred in part because the healthcare agencies believe they should receive payment for allowing their staff to educate students and partly because medical schools and some physician assistant programs pay for and compete with nursing schools for placements. It is difficult for public nursing programs to afford these placements and may lose placements to private and for-profit SON that may be better positioned to pay. In lieu of payment, public programs may seek other ways to show their clinical partners appreciation and to initiate or strengthen these relationships.

Excellent students and graduates are the best advertisements for a clinical agency to partner with an SON. Hospitals and other healthcare organizations get feedback from patients and visitors regarding the quality of care provided by students and employees. These organizations are looking for potential employees so the opportunity to get to know the quality of each student is beneficial to them.

Reminding clinical agencies that your program has a high board pass rate or that your students are superior to those from other schools— without appearing critical of other schools or programs—is perfectly acceptable because agencies can pick and choose the SON with which they would like to partner. Ultimately, it is in their best interest to provide clinical practice for students they would like to eventually hire. Convincing and reminding them that yours are the best is in your best interest. Flexibility to accommodate the needs of the agency and the expectation that they will take students from more than one SON is most likely to lead to good working relationships. Consider weekend and evening clinical practica and be willing to be creative about scheduling.

Immersion experiences whereby students spend a full semester in a particular setting on a specific unit allow both the student and the agency

Box 7.1 Keys to Developing and Strengthening Clinical Partnerships

- Flexibility
- Immersion/internship experiences
- Board of visitors
- Partnership council or committee
- Joint appointment models
- Awards and events that involve partners and alumni
- Regular communication via meetings with chief nursing officers

to get to know each other and whether they want to pursue employment after graduation. Immersion experiences allow students to experience what it would be like to be a nurse in a specific setting by working one on one with a preceptor, including working the shifts the preceptor works. There is time to get to know the organization as the student is getting all of his or her clinical experience in one setting for an entire semester. By the end of the semester, the student has received a solid orientation and, if hired, can "hit the ground running."

Employment of graduates is a surefire way to ensure that alumni will support clinical placements for students and continued employment of new graduates. Including chief nursing officers on a board of visitors or advisory board of the SON can also help ensure continued goodwill. Quarterly meetings at the SON, in which the board members hear the latest news and can share what they consider qualifications of prospective employees, can meet the needs of both the SON and the clinical partners. This can also be accomplished by inviting the staff nurses and agency staff educators to an annual meeting with faculty to share ideas and suggestions.

Joint appointments are another excellent mechanism for strengthening partnerships and can also save money for the SON. There are a variety of models for this and each one can be individualized further, according to the needs of the SON and the clinical partner agency. Public universities cannot pay outside agencies for employees; however, the clinical partner agency can pay the public university SON to share the cost of salaries and fringe benefits for shared employees.

Examples of models include sharing a faculty researcher who can conduct research for and within the clinical agency while on faculty. In this model, the faculty may have credits paid for by the clinical agency to perform research for them. It is ideal for the faculty to be able to then publish and otherwise disseminate that research. A clinical agency might consider an endowed professorship whereby they fund the faculty line for a period of 3 to 5 years and in return get to name the professorship and have the endowed professor work on their projects.

Another example is that of the advanced practice registered nurse (APRN) who is employed as faculty for the SON but who also has a joint clinical appointment in the clinical partner agency. The APRN faculty may also assist the partner agency with evidence-based-practice projects or other clinical initiatives. The other most common type of joint appointment is a shared clinical placement. In this model, an RN employed by the clinical partner agency teaches clinical practica for the SON without additional pay from the SON. This master's- or doctorally prepared nurse may sit on SON committees and engage in SON activities and acts as a liaison with the clinical partner agency to acquire clinical experiences and opportunities for students. This nurse may also help develop and conduct nurse residency programs and orientations for the agency and initiate and guide quality-improvement projects. This model goes beyond the RN who is employed at a clinical agency and teaches a clinical or two for the SON. There is typically equal responsibility for paying the salary and benefits for this nurse and a structured plan for the work she or he will do for each organization.

Awards and award events for exceptional clinical nurses who work in the partner agencies are other excellent ways of showing the partner agencies how much they are valued by the SON. The SON might sponsor an annual fund-raising event to recognize exceptional clinical nurses from throughout the region and ask clinical partner agencies to purchase tables for their employees to attend.

Attending agency events on behalf of the SON is an effective way to demonstrate interest in the community and in the goals of the partner organizations. Inviting agencies to SON events often results in reciprocal invitations to participate in agency events. The SON should take advantage of every possible opportunity to engage the agencies.

Partner agencies in which SON alumni are employed may be willing to host alumni events. The academic nurse leader can work with the SON advancement officer to organize these events. These are excellent opportunities for the SON to encourage agency employees to return to their alma mater for continued education. These events also serve the clinical agency by demonstrating their support for continuing education and the partnership with the SON.

SON that are part of academic health centers may find it easier to collaborate with clinical partners because there is an inherent relationship; however, these also must be nourished and continually strengthened. New ideas and innovative ways to engage students and clinicians will help enhance clinical experiences for students and ensure placements in the future.

Frequent and regular communication with clinical partners is key. The academic nurse leader should arrange regular meetings—about once a semester—with the chief nurse executive (CNE) of each of the larger healthcare organizations with which they partner. This one-on-one interaction reminds the CNE of how highly you value them and their organization and demonstrates a willingness to listen to their suggestions and concerns.

Establishing new programs often requires contracting with agencies to provide student experiences as part of the accrediting process. This author experienced this when developing a nurse anesthesia program. She and her program director made frequent visits to hospitals and surgical centers to educate the staff about the program and how the partnership would enable nurses to obtain the certification for nurse anesthesia rather than leave the state to seek it elsewhere. Conversations to discuss details and allay concerns may need to be repeated as everyone begins to understand the role each will play.

International partnerships are an excellent way to increase clinical placements while also giving students the opportunity of a lifetime. Most public universities have an office that handles international study or "study abroad." Get to know the people at that office and the services they provide. What are the options for student travel? Typically, there are many different configurations and variations in study-abroad opportunities.

Clinical experiences can take place during or between semesters or during a portion of the summer. It is possible to arrange a compressed clinical experience, in 2 to 3 weeks, for example, during which students care for patients in another country and also get opportunities for sightseeing and learning about the country. Partnering with a university that also has a SON is most helpful. So many possibilities can develop as a result. Students from both countries can take classes together, see patients together, and even work on research and other projects together. Relationships that begin during the study-abroad trip can continue via technology after students return to the United States.

Faculty typically enjoy these experiences as well because they are a break from the normal routine and they can be innovative about developing these experiences. Disadvantages include being away from their families for extended periods and staying with students all day every day.

It is helpful to assign a faculty member as the study-abroad coordinator for the SON. Remuneration can occur through a stipend or course credit. This faculty can work with the university's international studies office and become familiar with the paperwork and organizations involved. They can also cultivate long-term relationships with partners abroad. Deans and directors are wise to make the trip whenever possible to demonstrate dedication to the partnership and a willingness to collaborate. Gifts are often expected and can go along way toward good will.

Students and faculty should receive the appropriate orientation and preparation for the trip. Students should be in excellent academic standing prior to traveling because they may not have time to study while away. Semester-long trips abroad will involve taking courses for credit and abiding by rules with which they will be unfamiliar. Being well prepared will help students and faculty to get the most out of the experience.

Encourage faculty members to be innovative as they plan these trips and once they are in the other country. For example, this author knows of a faculty member who created a children's library associated with the hospital abroad because she learned they did not have one. Donations of nursing texts are commonplace, especially to SON in countries that cannot afford to buy the texts we have. Consider also clinical experiences in the United States in underserved areas, such as on Native American communities and in underserved areas.

Faculty Practice

It is this author's bias that faculty who engage in some form of their own practice outside of teaching are better prepared to educate nurses about the realities of the clinical environment. Faculty practice does not necessarily mean that the faculty is providing direct patient care. If the faculty has a specialty in nursing administration and teaches nursing leadership, then perhaps a greater presence on hospital executive boards than other faculty might be the expectation. However, nurse educators who teach clinical courses should be able to speak intelligently about current practice. The ability to do so gives them credibility with students and may ultimately enhance NCLEX® pass rates because students learn what is happening in practice rather than extrapolating from books or online resources.

In some SON, non-advanced-practice registered nursing faculty might practice throughout the academic year or during holiday and summer vacations. Sometimes, the interest a faculty member has in working clinically can be negotiated into a joint appointment with a healthcare organization.

Public universities frequently require all faculty to sign a form disclosing any work they perform outside the university. It can be a cause for concern when someone works for the public university and another state agency. However, the faculty is required to reveal all sources of outside income, including consultation work.

The SON will choose how to handle faculty practice based on its resources and whether the SON can financially support faculty taking 1 day per week or other time off of work to engage in clinical practice. Some universities require that the faculty be paid through the university. In other words, the clinical site pays the university for "borrowing" the faculty and the faculty gets remunerated by having the faculty practice time count toward his or her workload. Other arrangements allow faculty to get paid directly by the clinical agency above and beyond their university salary. In those cases, nurse academic leaders should help faculty understand that the SON is paying them even on days they are working elsewhere and getting paid by another organization, especially when resources are scarce and it is necessary to negotiate faculty workload.

■ THE FOR-PROFIT UNIVERSITY PERSPECTIVE

The number of direct care clinical hours required for a program is determined by the state board of nursing and varies widely. Multistate programs that have a centralized syllabus and set of graduation requirements must default to the highest number required in order to satisfy all state board regulations. In most states, a new school must prove that there are sufficient clinical agency experiences available for the planned enrollment prior to opening. This is a tremendous challenge facing the proprietary sector, which has grown exponentially over the past decade (Baum, Kurose, & McPherson, 2013). This growth has increased the pressure on already overextended clinical partners to provide the number of clinical spaces needed to support that growth. Many states are saturated with nursing programs and may be denying requests for opening new schools based on the lack of clinical spaces, especially those states with high clinical hour requirements.

According to the National League for Nursing (2014), the number of nursing programs across the United States exceeds 1,800. Many for-profit organizations that have opened nursing programs in the last decade find themselves competing with programs that have long-standing relationships with clinical partners and as a result may be denied space or offered space on nights and weekends that are hard to staff and may not offer the best experience for students. In order to treat all schools fairly, some healthcare organizations have started using a lottery system for awarding clinical slots. This practice makes it exceedingly difficult to plan schedules in advance, which, in turn, leads to student dissatisfaction. Although all program types aim for student satisfaction, in the for-profit sector, student satisfaction ratings may be used as performance measures for the leadership team and, in some organizations, are part of the faculty evaluation as well. Given the challenges facing the for-profit sector, the clinical coordinator should have charisma and excellent "soft skills" like professionalism, relationship building, negotiating, and interpersonal communication. On more than one occasion, it has been the relationship between the clinical coordinator and the educational liaison at the agency that resulted in getting the desperately needed additional clinical space.

Clinical coordination is one of the more stressful jobs in the nursing program as clinical practica are critical to meeting state regulations and program success. Losing a clinical coordinator can be devastating to a program so programs should take care in hiring for this position and meeting the personal and professional needs of the person in that role. It is wise to involve the clinical coordinator in scheduling as well as in the student-compliance process. All clinical partners require nursing programs to verify that students have taken a cardiopulmonary resuscitation (CPR) course, have current immunizations, and background checks prior to starting clinical. The clinical coordinator may be responsible for maintaining these student records and sending attestation forms to the clinical partners or they may work with a compliance team. Large multistate programs tend to have centralized compliance departments, which can be a benefit or a drawback depending on how well the clinical coordinator and compliance team work together.

Many states have approved the use of simulation to ease the pressure on clinical agencies. Once again, each state has rules about the percentage of clinical hours that can be completed by simulation. This allowance can be found in the state regulations and can vary from 15% to 50% of total clinical hours. There may be regulations related to the percentage by course as well as the overall percentage of simulated hours allowed. Multistate programs will again set a percentage that meets the requirements of its most stringent state. Proprietary programs tend to have exquisitely appointed simulation labs as they tend to have more financial resources that can be applied to simulation labs and equipment, can develop partnerships with vendors that result in cost savings due to the number of campuses being served, and have more opportunity to modify or "build out" the physical plant.

Observational experiences are generally not allowed to be counted toward the direct-care hours required, but may be used in some cases to offset the differences between the program requirements for clinical hours, which may be higher than the direct-care hours required by the state.

In addition to the struggle to find clinical placements, all program types struggle to find qualified clinical faculty. Proprietary programs rely on adjuncts for clinical education, although some do hire full-time clinical faculty, especially in high-demand areas such as psychiatric and pediatric nursing. Adjuncts should be oriented to the values and expectations of the nursing program and the unit/agency to which they are assigned. Because adjunct faculty are limited by the Department of Education in the number of hours they can work for any given school, they often work for a number of programs at the same time. You want to be sure they are following your model of supervision. Some colleges have resorted to using employment agencies to staff clinicals. Although this may be necessary in the short term, it places the program at increased risk and generally costs 25% more per hour than the standard pay. Clinical faculty can make or break a program as they are the face of the program in the agency. Placements have been lost because of the attitude or demeanor of the clinical faculty. On the positive side, but equally problematic, some facilities like an instructor so much they only want that person on the unit. Visiting the units at least once a term ensures that both the agency and the student needs are being met and strengthens the relationship with the school, not just the clinical faculty.

Terms in most proprietary programs run anywhere from 5 to 10 weeks without any breaks between terms, which is both a benefit and a drawback. On the plus side, shorter terms increase the adjunct pool as it offers faculty more flexibility and opportunity. The drawback is that the leadership team is constantly hiring and orienting adjuncts to be sure that the supply is sufficient each term.

The use of joint appointments is not common in the for-profit sector although many nursing programs are looking at establishing dedicated educational units with consistent faculty oversight that have the potential to evolve to a joint appointment. Similarly, nursing programs that utilize unpaid agency preceptors have opportunities to offer those preceptors faculty appointments or other perquisites that benefit all parties and open doors for increased sharing of clinical resources.

One way to develop new partnerships is through career fairs. Most for-profit schools have a career services department dedicated to helping students apply for and secure employment. These departments bring a variety of healthcare agencies to campus several times a year and allow them to speak to the students about opportunities for employment and externships and set up interviews. This is an excellent time for the campus leadership to connect personally with the visiting team and asking about opportunities for student experiences. If the owner, director, or education liaison is not present, getting their contact information personally and following up with a phone call that begins, "I got your card from . . ." can open doors that would not have opened by "cold calling."

Another avenue available to for-profits is the advisory board. Nursing program advisory boards in the for-profit sector are generally made up of agencies that employ graduates of the program. This is because the board's purpose is to advise the program about the quality of the graduates from their very real-world experience with them. Making the board members aware of the need for clinical sites can lead to increased placements with the board member agencies themselves or referrals to other partners such as outpatient clinics, hospice facilities, and prisons. Participating on professional boards yourself or on state and national committees can also open up opportunities by increasing your network. Sharing resources can be mutually beneficial. For example, you can grant partners access to simulation labs for staff development in exchange for use of clinical space at their facility.

Another collaborative opportunity being explored in the proprietary sector is partnering with a specific hospital or healthcare system with the intention of making hiring decisions in the student's final semester so that the student is being oriented to the facility as they are completing their final practicum. This helps the agency reduce orientation costs and secures a high-quality, one-to-one precepted internship practicum, which is increasingly difficult to obtain. This requires matching students with units and organizations and allowing agencies to select which students they will take into the advanced hiring program, but it is an attractive option that has the potential to increase placements, decrease costs, and help students transition to practice.

Equal to securing placements is keeping them. Clinical placements are always at risk. Nursing staff can see the students as creating work and being in the way or as an asset. They can be excited about the opportunity to teach or they can feel resentful that they have to stop their work to teach nursing students. Developing a positive relationship with the unit nurses is the responsibility of the clinical instructor. Establishing trust and credibility is the first step in this process. The best scenario is hiring clinical faculty who are known to the agency, but if that is not possible, the unit orientation should be used to demonstrate clinical acumen and willingness to support the unit nurses and their routines. When there is a good fit between instructor and unit staff, the instructor is viewed as part of the team and students move through the unit seamlessly. How students behave on the units is critical to maintaining placements and cannot be overstated. For-profit schools tend to admit students from disadvantaged backgrounds who may not have developed interpersonal skills or understand professional conduct at the level expected by clinical partners. It pays to be very explicit with instructions about dress (down to the detail of clean and unwrinkled uniforms), arrival time, conversation on the unit, parking, use of the conference room, and so on. This author is aware of a program that lost a clinical site because the nurse manager overheard a student complaining about having to pass out medications. It is interesting to note that student mistakes are generally taken in stride, usually it is the small infractions like parking in the wrong place or "standing around" that create the biggest reactions. Perhaps, this is because these actions appear deliberate and disrespectful. In reality, students may park in a wrong spot in order to be on time perceiving tardiness to be worse than violating a parking rule. Clinical orientation for students must be explicit and provide information not only about the rules, but also about the culture they are entering and the unit's values, especially in precepted clinical experiences, as the student is operating under the guidance of the agency RN with the school instructor on standby. See Box 7.2 for some considerations regarding keys to successful clinical management.

Box 7.2 Keys to Successful Clinical Management

- Obtaining sites
- Build relationships with agency partners
- Keeping sites
- Careful orientation of faculty
- Explicit instructions for students

(continued)

Box 7.2 Keys to Successful Clinical Management (*continued*)

- Respect nursing unit values and culture
- Ongoing relationship building with education liaison and nurse managers
- Keeping clinical faculty
- Visit clinical site to offer support
- Provide clear expectations for time on unit, student experiences, paperwork
- Demonstrate appreciation for challenges presented by the clinical site and reward loyalty

Faculty Practice

Many for-profit schools do not allow full-time faculty to work for other institutions. In those institutions where faculty are provided with a development day each week, it would be useful to have them working to keep their skills current. Not only does it enhance their teaching, it increases the likelihood that they will be able to step up and help out with clinical instruction should the need arise. In today's environment with heightened concern for safety, most healthcare organizations require clinical faculty to have 2 years of recent clinical experience in the specific clinical area assigned. Many classroom faculty could not meet this criterion. Linking clinical practice to faculty development and advising faculty upon hiring that they may be asked to do clinical teaching helps to maintain the supply of clinical-ready faculty.

■ THE PRIVATE UNIVERSITY PERSPECTIVE

A new nursing academic leader should become very familiar with all the faculty and staff in the SON and in the university, as we have addressed in other chapters. The next most important connection will be with nursing leaders at clinical agencies, especially if the nurse leader is moving to a new geographic area where there is not a familiarity with the clinical agencies with whom the school partners. The new nursing academic leader should set up individual meetings, if possible, to introduce yourself as a new SON leader and have both informal and formal conversations about aspects of your nursing program and the healthcare agency needs, which are outlined in Box 7.3.

It is a good practice to sustain and maintain relationships with nursing leaders from clinical agencies. This may include relationships with chief

Box 7.3 Topics to Discuss Between the SON Leader and Healthcare Agency Nursing Leader

Healthcare agency leader's perceptions of

- Reputation of the SON
- How students from the SON represent themselves during clinical experiences
- Strengths and deficits in graduates from the SON who have been hired into the agency
- Current and future healthcare trends and how they affect the profession of nursing
- Projected needs for nurses in the next 5 to 10 years at the organization

Academic leader's perceptions of

- Vision for the SON
- Proposed changes or enhancements to existing programs
- Curriculum and how it prepares graduates to practice nursing
- Current and future clinical needs
- Ideas for new programs

SON, school of nursing.

nurse officers, clinical placement coordinators, nurse educators, and even administrators such as the agency president. Healthcare agency leaders need a continual supply of nurses, and SON leaders need ongoing placements for clinical learning, so a mutually beneficial relationship should be established and continually nurtured.

For nursing education for all schools, clinical partnerships help supplement theoretical learning and expose students to professional nursing practice. Many schools and healthcare agencies have worked diligently in recent years to attempt to standardize processes and procedures for clinical requests and student placement requirements. Some states (e.g., Michigan and Oregon) or regions may require that all healthcare agencies and schools belong to a network, such as ACEMAPP™, which "is a secure, online, clinical rotation matching, student on-boarding, and document storage solution for clinical sites, schools and consortia" (https:// acemapp.org). Clinical requests are made within the ACEMAPP software program and healthcare agencies use the software to match the requests with the available spots within their organizations. Such software programs can also serve as the repository for students' health records and can include options for student, preceptor, clinical agency, and instructor evaluations. Some software programs include options for students to track their individual clinical experiences and reports can be generated that will help to show compliance with accreditation or regulatory standards. These software programs may add a cost to clinical placement that is often passed on to the students. However, streamlining and standardizing clinical-placement processes across multiple agencies and for all educational programs can save tremendous time and manual labor. This needs to be taken into consideration when appraising the associated costs and benefits.

Many academic nursing leaders and leaders from healthcare agencies have come together for both formal and informal partnerships that can strengthen clinical placement and nursing education in a city or region. In Wisconsin, for example, there are regional associations such as the Southeast Wisconsin Nursing Alliance (SEWNA), to which this author's school belongs. There are similar alliances for the northeast, northwest, and southwest regions in the state of Wisconsin. These alliances are made up of both clinical agency and nursing education leaders. The goal for SEWNA is to "advance and align nursing education and nursing practice through a community partnership of Southeastern Wisconsin healthcare systems and academic executive leadership" (www.wisconsincenterfornursing .org/anew-southeast.html). This goal is similar for all of the alliances in their respective regions. Members of these alliances have worked collaboratively to standardize students' health requirements and orientation processes for clinical placement, as well as processes and procedures for SON to secure clinical placements within the healthcare agencies. Typically, nursing leaders from the larger healthcare organizations within the region act as important members of these regional alliances, but it is impossible to have all healthcare agencies represented. Smaller organizations, such as long-term care facilities, transitional care services, dialysis centers, rehabilitation facilities, public health agencies, schools, and other community agencies, are often not represented. Therefore, 100% standardization is not probable and individual variations for clinical requirements and placements will occur, especially with smaller healthcare agencies and transitional care services.

Clinical agencies deal with a plethora of requests for clinical placement each semester: clinical groups; one-on-one precepted experiences with RNs and advanced practice nurses; and shadowing opportunities to observe nursing practice in a specific setting are made each semester from local, regional, and other SON. Clinical agencies include acute and long-term care agencies, community settings, home care agencies, public health departments, and a multitude of transitional care areas that are becoming more and more typical sites for healthcare delivery. Agencies receive requests from local, regional, and national traditional prelicensure programs; accelerated prelicensure programs; postlicensure programs (BSN completion); and advanced practice programs that include students in both master's- and doctoral-level programs. Requests can come from more traditional programs with on-the-ground campuses (brick and mortar) or from online programs.

Healthcare agencies have the ultimate ability to accept or deny requests for clinical placement. Some agencies have rules or guidelines in place addressing to whom they may give priority placement. For example, if a nurse is working at an organization and is enrolled in an educational program leading to a degree or an advanced degree in nursing, the clinical agency may "guarantee" placement for that nurse in the hopes of keeping a good employee within the same organization after graduation even if it is into a different role. Therefore, student nurses in a traditional undergraduate program may be successfully placed into a precepted clinical practicum within the organization in which they work. This is mutually beneficial to the students and the organization and clinical placement coordinators should capitalize on such opportunities.

Some SON may have their own "rules" that students working within an organization should be encouraged to complete clinical experiences in a different organization to add to their depth of exposure to varied settings. However, leaders at SON need to explore these types of "rules" carefully to see whether there is evidence to support such a practice. They should assess individual students' professional objectives; if students are hoping to be hired within that same organization in which they are currently working after graduation, it seems counterintuitive to require them to have clinical placements in a different organization. Having students stay within the same organization could potentially decrease the orientation time as a student (they may already be familiar with the computer systems and policies and procedures) as well as the orientation time once hired into the new role. This familiarity can save the healthcare organization time and money. Some healthcare agencies guarantee jobs to those employees who choose to continue their education to become an RN or an advanced practice nurse. Therefore, keeping them within the organization makes the most sense, as long as the healthcare organization has the capability of offering all the clinical learning experiences required by the program. Students within all levels of nursing programs must understand that during clinical experiences, they are acting within the role and scope of a student nurse, not as an employee. For example, a student in prelicensure nursing program would be acting in the role of the student RN, not in the role of a certified nursing assistant, surgical technologist, or licensed practical nurse, and those role expectations need to be clear during all clinical learning experiences.

Some healthcare organizations have developed policies for accepting or not accepting students from online programs. These policies should similarly be closely reviewed as they may represent an unfounded bias that online programs are not as successful in educating nurses as those that offer face-to-face courses. Healthcare leaders should understand that program delivery methods do not necessarily equate with its students' success or lack thereof. It is the quality of the program, including its curriculum, admission, and progression criteria, and the quality of the faculty who teach in the program that have the greatest influence on students' and the program's success or failure, and not the mode of delivering the curriculum and its components.

Private schools typically have higher tuition rates than their public counterparts. "Selling" their programs to potential students typically focuses on the value that students receive in exchange for that higher tuition. Refer to Chapter 6 (marketing) for specific strategies used to share that message clearly and widely. Private schools can highlight their unique student and curricular characteristics to agency leaders. Sometimes healthcare agency leaders will note that graduates from private universities are desired over those from other schools because of their professionalism and character. Agency leaders may note that graduates from private schools are not only prepared clinically and theoretically, but they may be more confident and caring with a strong commitment to living the private university's mission and showing they are well prepared for their vocation as a professional nurse.

Private schools can often connect clinical learning with their mission. For example, they may have opportunities for students to provide healthcare in underserved areas locally, regionally, or globally. These types of trips may connect healing with faith and/or spreading the university's mission to others. Often, these experiences can be tied to clinical learning in which a student would have experiences that could meet clinical course objectives while on the trip. Sometimes, the university or a religious-affiliated organization may provide scholarships to support students in serving in such work, making it very appealing for students to participate in such activities. Nurse educators have to be sure that the work on the trip is beyond observational, which often cannot be counted toward clinical hours. However, nurse educators can work carefully to ensure that experiences during trips are action oriented and meet clinical learning objectives. Nurse leaders must take into account that clinical experiences such as those obtained during such trips still need to comply with the state's board of nursing and accreditation requirements for aspects such as the qualifications necessary for those providing supervision.

Students who have participated in such trips and global experiences in which they were able to perform clinical practice have found them to be life changing. The immersion in the culture helps them to identify the socioeconomic and health disparities across the globe. Experiencing healthcare systems in which patients and families must pay for medications and services or be denied treatment, to work in facilities in which the technology is vastly behind that available in the United States or in places in which electricity may be a luxury, or to provide care in areas and situations in which the poor are even more underserved than in the United States are examples of conditions that can provoke very emotional reactions. Such clinical experiences can be triggers for students to commit to lifelong service or community service work related to local, regional, and global initiatives to improve health and health outcomes.

Using nontraditional sites that may not be used by competing schools is another means for private schools to capitalize on clinical learning opportunities. For example, a faith-based school may offer community or transitional care clinical practica in a parish or congregational setting. Often these have to be one-on-one precepted experiences, because even large congregations are fortunate if they have one or two nurses acting as congregational nurses. Such an experience exposes students to a nursing specialty of which they may not be aware. Similarly, although public, for-profit, and private universities may offer community or pediatric clinical rotations within public school systems, private SON may have a unique connection with private grade schools or high schools with which they may share an affiliation.

As noted earlier, using clinical agencies during "off" times can be a benefit to programs in securing placements that may otherwise be taken up by competing schools. Private schools can often be nimbler in revising academic or university policies to make completing clinical practica during off times a reasonable alternative for students. For example, a policy change regarding traditional semesters and associated tuition requirements could make it possible for students to have clinical during the summer months as part of their spring or fall semester academic load and without paying additional summer school tuition. This would allow clinical experiences at summer camps or at acute care agencies using a more immersive style in which students could attend clinical for 2 to 3 weeks in a row Monday through Friday rather than attending 1 day per week for an entire semester. This type of immersion experience allows students to follow patients over time and to be exposed to the continuity of patient care they may not see during a more traditional 1-day-per-week clinical offering.

Interprofessional clinical education is rapidly gaining favor so that students of different disciplines can learn together in a clinical setting to provide patient-centered care and prepare them to work as team members, which will be expected after graduation. Dedicated education units are often used for this purpose in acute settings. However, interprofessional clinical education should be expanded to more nontraditional settings such as community mental health agencies, rehabilitation clinics, and drug rehabilitation programs. Interprofessional clinical education can pose challenges for supervision as each discipline has individual regulations regarding appropriate clinical oversight for students in their respective professions. For example, for an interprofessional student team consisting of nursing, physical therapy, occupational therapy, and pharmacy students to provide care in a community-based setting, faculty members from each discipline may also be required to provide direct supervision or oversight. This can make implementing such clinical experiences a challenge. This author believes that as interprofessional education becomes more and more prominent in preparing students for the work that will be expected of them after graduation, accrediting and regulating bodies will have to reexamine their policies on oversight requirements to make interprofessional clinical education easier to operationalize.

High-ranking nursing leaders should act as part of the SON's advisory council (referred to in the section on public perspectives as the "Board of Visitors") so that input and planning regarding current and future clinical learning needs for various programs are discussed in an ongoing manner and support can be gained and maintained for the school and its programs. Although the high-level leaders are not the ones actually facilitating clinical placements within their organizations, their approval and ongoing support makes such agreements happen. At this author's university, we invited each member of our advisory council to either personally participate or send a representative to spend one entire day on campus to review the curriculum and gain working professional nurses' input into our traditional undergraduate program curriculum. From their input, we learned that we needed much more emphasis on pediatric mental health and on having our students in more transitional care areas as opposed to the current emphasis on clinical practica in acute care agencies. We also gained input from agency leaders to support preceptorships in both acute and community settings. We appreciated the advisory council allowing their staff a full day away from work to provide this input to improve our curriculum.

As part of the clinical agency–SON alignment, private schools can sometimes offer incentives, such as tuition discounts, to nurses working at the healthcare agencies with which the SON has clinical contracts. Tuition discounts could be offered for various reasons. For example, if a certain number of associate degree-prepared nurses are working at a specific healthcare agency or within facilities in its system, and they are willing to commit to entering a private school's BSN completion program, a tuition discount might be applied for that group. Such agreements and discounts can make private school tuition more in line with that of public universities. Leaders at healthcare agencies may be less inclined to sign "exclusive" agreements with any one academic institution, especially with a private university. The foundational tenets of a private school may conflict with those of the public (or even private) healthcare organization. Yet such agreements and discounts will allow nurses who work at those organizations to choose a private school to begin or continue their education without incurring significantly additional tuition costs as compared to a public university.

Faculty Practice

At private universities, guidelines and expectations for faculty practice are similar to those described for public universities. The one unique aspect is that faculty within private organizations may regularly engage in practice on service trips or within other service agencies. Faculty may provide healthcare in developing countries, in areas of need in the United States, or in free clinics that may or may not be affiliated with the university. Although this type of practice may not be for pay, it may help faculty to fulfill a service component expected for advancement in rank or to achieve tenure. Often, faculty can engage and oversee students in these endeavors, which help to promote the university's mission, and also allows students to provide patient-centered care in more challenging settings than they may see in their traditional clinical rotations.

REFERENCES

Baum, S., Kurose, C., & McPherson, M. (2013). An overview of American higher education. *Future of Children, 23*(1), 17–39.

Boyer, E. L. (1990). *Scholarship reconsidered*. San Francisco, CA: Jossey-Bass.

National League for Nursing. (2014). Annual survey of schools of nursing, academic year 2013–2014. Retrieved from http://www.nln.org/newsroom/nursing-education-statistics/annual-survey-of-schools-of-nursing-academic-year-2013–2014

CHAPTER 8

ALLOCATION AND UTILIZATION OF RESOURCES

Budgeting and the allocation of resources are key components of the role of the dean. Schools of nursing (SON) will vary widely regarding how much budget management support is provided to the nurse academic leader. In addition, there is a wide variety of budget models and each one has inherent advantages, disadvantages, and risks. Faculty may be more or less involved in budget-related decisions depending on their roles. Faculty in leadership positions, such as chairs, directors, assistant, or associate deans, may manage their own budgets. The aspiring nurse academic leader should devote some time to learning about typical budget models used in higher education.

■ THE PUBLIC UNIVERSITY PERSPECTIVE

Budgeting in a public university is challenging. "Beyond mission confusion, the financing of public universities appears to be a mystery to many" (Fethke & Policano, 2012, p. 67). The state provides most of the funding for the public university. The idea of a public university is to make college affordable to citizens, so tuition tends to be lower than that for private or for-profit universities. Not infrequently, the state may decide to lower public university tuition or abandon it altogether. In addition to tuition, fees, and state funding, the public university may receive monies through federal loans, grants, donations, and selling its services.

Public universities are typically bound by specific rules and policies that are intended to safeguard public funding. Consequently, public universities are limited as to what they can pay for, how they can pay for it, and how much they can pay. For example, on a small scale, there may be rules about paying for lunch during a meeting. The meeting may have to last most of the day and extend through a normal mealtime to qualify. On a larger scale, public money may be restricted with regard to renovating and building facilities.

To some degree, the mission of the university drives the amount of money the university receives and from whom (Fethke & Policano, 2012). For example, a public university whose primary mission is research will receive much more grant funding and endowments than the nonresearch public university. If sports is a major function of the university, then much of the funding it receives (and its costs) will be related to athletics.

The politics of the state and the Board of Trustees or Regents significantly influence how valued the public universities are both financially and educationally. For example, in Wisconsin, funding for the public universities has steadily declined, whereas funding for technical (community) colleges has continued to rise. This is a reflection of the value the state places on jobs, rather than on professions or learning for learning's sake. Frequent and lasting tuition freezes tie the hands of university administrators who continue to strive to offer quality education and retain exceptional faculty and staff.

Public universities are intended to provide education to the public and must make allowances for those in need. Many states have reduced tuition or eliminated it altogether. Legislators have reduced their support for higher education but still require public universities to decrease tuition for needy students and to accept community college students through articulation agreements. These policies further reduce revenue for public universities (Fethke & Policano, 2012).

Money that is allocated from the state specifically for salaries and fringe benefits cannot typically be used to pay for anything else. The university usually has other program revenue, frequently generated by the schools or colleges within the university, to help subsidize faculty salaries and benefits and strategic initiatives. For example, program revenue in the SON might come from the doctorate in nursing practice (DNP) program. Salaries and benefits for faculty teaching in the DNP program might come from the DNP account.

Although there are several different budget models (Table 8.1) the university might choose to use, philosophically, if not in actual practice, public universities have cost centers and revenue centers. The SON is an example of a revenue center because it brings in tuition, but it is also mainly supported

Table 8.1 Examples of Budget Models Used in Higher Education

Budget Model	Explanation
Incremental budget management	This is a centralized approach that relies on data from the previous year. Allocations are not likely to change significantly from year to year.
Incentive-based budget management	This is a decentralized approach whose most popular models are activity-based management and responsibility-centered management. It tends to be very transparent and allow for a large degree of unit autonomy.
Performance-based budget management	This is a centralized to semicentralized approach that uses performance targets on which to base allocations.
Formula-based budget management	This is a centralized approach that uses formulas to determine needs and allocations.
Zero-based budget management	This is a centralized approach in which the budget is zeroed at the end of each year and the unit must justify a new budget every year.

by tuition. Dining services is also a revenue center but it is supported by its own fees and is likely to also be supported by fees the students pay in addition to their tuition (sometimes called *segregated fees*). The revenue centers are taxed in some way to help support central administration ("central") or the university administration, which then helps pay the cost centers or are taxed directly by the cost centers for their services. Depending on the budget model used by the university, each center may be allocated a certain amount of money from the tuition and state subsidy based on whatever measure is determined by their governance structure or they may receive all of their tuition and revenue but have to pay a larger bill for the services they use. University units, such as the SON, might not "see" the tuition they earn but are simply allotted an amount of money that is already minus the amount "central" has decided to subtract to pay for university services to the unit.

Cost centers are generally university departments that do not bring in revenue, such as human resources or the provost's office. These centers must rely on the revenue centers to fund them, either via a central tax to the university or by a fee-for-service system. This fee-for-service system might be determined based on the number of full-time equivalents (FTEs) the revenue unit has. For example, in the case of Human

Resources, if the SON has 30 faculty, 10 adjunct faculty, and six clerical staff, and all are 1.0 FTE (full-time equivalent), then the SON might pay a percentage to human resources based on 46 FTE. Human Resources has to perform work for all faculty and staff in the university so this makes sense. However, the SON may pay the library based on student credit hours rather than employee FTE because students are more likely to use the library than are faculty and staff. The provost's office only serves those in academic affairs. Consequently, not all revenue units will fund the provost's office. Again, depending on the budget model used, the university may initially subtract a specified amount to go toward university services before allocating the budget to the unit.

In other areas, such as the student health clinic, students may pay a special fee as part of their tuition in addition to a fee-for-service arrangement. The special student fee that is part of tuition may also pay for student clubs and help subsidize residence halls.

Faculty may receive block grants (money from the state via the university) or revenue from other internal sources (such as a dean's new investigator grant) to support their research. They may also apply for funding from external federal or private grant sources. *Indirect funding*, when the term is used with regard to external grants, refers to overhead that is included in the research grant budget, such as funding to support a portion of the faculty member's time to work on the research study or to support the use of a laboratory or other university resources during the research study.

Public universities that are research universities may operate somewhat differently from other public universities. When there is a decline in research funding, faculty may be required to teach more. If demand for classes changes or the subsidy from the state declines, fewer faculty researchers may be hired with a subsequent decline in funded research. Alternative methods of instruction are more likely to appear. Much support has shifted to teaching and away from research due to public demand and declining enrollment. It is hard to justify course releases to support research when students are paying more or there is a decline in public support. This has led to a decrease in tenure-track, faculty researchers. Substitution with part-time or nondoctorally prepared faculty may reduce instructional quality. In addition, the new presidential administration has indicated it is less supportive of higher education and of grant funding for academic research.

Budget Models

Typically, a budget model is either centralized or decentralized. In the former, the university (chancellor/president or his or her designee) determines the allocations to the schools/colleges/units. In the latter, the units make the most of their choices about how to generate revenue and pay costs. They pay a percentage based on a variety of possible parameters to the university to help the university fund its own operations and those of units that do not generate revenue.

Public universities have a habit of "sweeping" funds from their schools and colleges when the university has bills it cannot pay. In the end, the university can do what it likes with "your" money; however, allocating money into budget lines that support the SON can help university administrators see that money is not just waiting to be swept away, but is allocated for important activities. For example, you might consider allocating some program revenue, if in alignment with university policy, into budget lines for professional development for faculty and staff. Very often, support staff do not get to go to professional development conferences and they, too, need and appreciate these opportunities. Some money might go into advertising or marketing (such as purchasing "swag" like pens or bags with the SON logo; see Chapter 6) or into a new investigator award for new faculty just beginning their programs of research.

The chief nursing administrator in a public SON tends to have a lot of discretion over budgetary matters. There typically is some flexibility in moving money between and among budget lines with the exception of state funding. State funding from tuition and tax dollars is usually specifically designated for salaries and fringe benefits. Student segregated fees are specifically designated as are other categories of funding. Budget lines that you create and to which you allocate are more fluid. You can move money from the line you designated for advertising to the line you created for professional development, for example. Typically, some salaries and fringe benefits can be drawn from program revenue to pay faculty who teach in those programs that produced the revenue.

If you are fortunate enough to have a budget analyst in the SON, work closely with the analyst and get to know how this person thinks. First, learn specifically for what the analyst is responsible. Is his or her main function to enter data pertaining to the budget and develop reports for the SON administrator and the university financial office? Does he or she have human resources functions, such as employee contracts? Has the analyst been given other responsibilities, such as approving the purchase of computer equipment, other technology, or lab supplies?

Also, meet with the university financial/budget office and preferably the chief budget officer (CBO) to learn what, if any, checks and balances exist. In other words, how can you, as the SON administrator, check to be sure that what your budget analyst records and reports is accurate? You should not begin your role suspicious of the person who will probably end up being one of your closest allies, but, as chief executive of the SON, you are responsible for the SON budget so you must know how you can ensure its accuracy. If there are inaccuracies or gaps, you will be held responsible, so getting to know your budget analyst and your budget can help avoid problems.

Some public universities are analyzing whether to change their budget models based on the changing landscape of support for public higher education. Many public institutions are experiencing a decline in state funding reflective of the decrease in the perceived value of higher education and other priorities for tax dollars. Repetitive tuition freezes and declines in tuition rob universities of the funding they require to pay faculty and staff salaries or reward merit. A decline in enrollment, particularly because there are fewer high school graduates and fewer of these apply to college, also erodes funding. University budget reductions may not be apparent to faculty and staff until they begin to impact their jobs, salaries, and the resources they need to perform their work; however, administrators must constantly be aware of the financial health of the university and the SON and plan ahead.

Challenges

An academic administrator should be able to predict budget implications. If the administrator can put mechanisms in place that will help the SON weather budget cuts, then faculty and staff are likely to be less disrupted by the reductions. However, the SON administrator walks a fine line. Although administrators should be transparent, faculty and staff who have not previously been exposed to academic budget matters may find the subject confusing and disturbing. Find out how much the faculty and staff already know, if anything, and try to determine how much, if anything, they would like to know. For example, this author served as dean at an SON that was not previously exposed to budget matters. The previous dean and budget analyst took care of everything associated with budgeting. Faculty told this author that they would like to know more about the budget and have some control over departmental budgets. That and a huge budget reduction enforced by the state system were the impetus for sharing budget details with the SON.

What this author did not foresee was the complexity of the public university system and the university budget model and that faculty and staff would become more confused rather than appreciate the transparency of knowing more about the budgeting process. Also, in their efforts to cope with and manage frequent and significant budget cuts and maintain quality, higher level administration at the university frequently changed their messages about the budget cuts and how the schools within the university should handle them. Further, higher level administration tried to maintain and raise employee morale so did not share how dire the budget situation really was. Consequently, this author's efforts to be transparent with faculty and staff were sometimes met with skepticism because of the mixed messages and the frequent changes to the bottom line.

Add to this that state legislators began to require that faculty account for all of their teaching time and demonstrate that they were teaching as many hours and for as many credits as expected by legislators and the public. This author tried to help faculty prepare for this expectation and for future budget cuts by ensuring that workload was distributed appropriately and that there could be no question regarding how faculty used their time to teach, conduct research, and engage in clinical practice. Some faculty resented the removal of course releases that had not resulted in scholarly deliverables or projects. Changing the mind-set from how things were done when resources were more plentiful and there was less scrutiny and accountability from legislators and the public to a new mind-set of clearly demonstrating the value of faculty work was incredibly challenging.

Despite this experience, the author believes that one should be transparent with faculty and staff about the budget, but with caveats. One can overwhelm faculty and staff if they are not assisted in developing a gradual and comprehensive understanding of how the budget model works before learning to interpret the budget itself. One should not take for granted that because people manage their household budgets or may have managed budgets in the clinical setting that they will understand an academic budget, especially one from a public university. It is also wise to educate your leadership team first so they can advocate for you when you begin to share aspects of the budget with the entire school. Be prepared for confusion and questions, in any case. It is risky to share the budget, not just because of concerns about the numbers themselves but because faculty and staff will not immediately understand all of the complexities and nuances that impact or are impacted by the budget. They cannot possibly comprehend these nuances unless they are privy to much of the other information to which the SON administrator is exposed in the normal business of the university so *proceed with caution*.

Perhaps begin by sharing the implications of the budget reductions and the foundations of how the budget model and process work at your university and within the public university system and later amplify this foundation by sharing budget lines and the actual numbers involved. Each SON administrator will find his or her own best way to proceed. We all want to be as transparent as possible but faculty and staff also have enough on their plates, so carefully weigh how much knowledge about the budget will serve to enlighten them and help them advise you and how much crosses the line into worrying them when things may swiftly change again.

The Impact of Shared Governance

The tenet of shared governance in public universities also impacts budgeting. Fethke and Policano (2012) contend that the most valued faculty are the least likely to serve on faculty senates because the most valued faculty are too busy with their own work and research to engage with the work of the senate. Johnson and Turner (2009) echo that those serving on the senate are more likely to gain from resisting new ideas. I do not necessarily agree; I have served on faculty senates because I wanted to be involved and because I cared about the future of the university. However, faculty have been known to resist new ideas just to resist and also because they are skeptical of the motivation behind administrator's actions. "A sobering reality is that the most likely reward for anyone who proposes strategic, innovative change that involves trade-offs is a short tenure in office" (Fethke & Policano, 2012, p. 177). A smart administrator learns to trust very few people and only those who have proven they can be trusted. It is also helpful to remember that higher administration, such as provosts and presidents, want to maintain morale and may give different messages about the state of the university to faculty and staff than those they give to deans and department heads.

Shared governance, particularly peer review and tenure, can help instill and maintain quality but is only truly effective when funding is available and likely to continue at a reasonable level. However, when resources are scarce and the environment is changing, governance that requires extensive and elaborate processes of approval can impede progress. Difficult choices, such as eliminating or reducing programs or removing course releases that do not contribute to enhancing research or revenue, will not sit well with faculty. "Even when planning works well and identifies promising areas, the governance process can stymie good ideas" (Fethke & Policano, 2012, p. 180).

As discussed elsewhere in this book, shared governance can be wonderful and informative and in its most idealistic version allows everyone to provide input and perspective. However, in practice, remember that the lengthy and sometimes convoluted processes inherent in shared governance can slow or prevent change. The wise SON administrator will value shared governance but also try to analyze its probable consequences before suggesting a new strategy or innovation, particularly one with budget implications.

Discretionary Funds

The degree of autonomy and latitude the chief nurse executive (CNE) has over the SON budget varies; however, in a public university, the CNE usually has a discretionary budget that can be used for whatever the CNE deems appropriate. A large portion, if not the total amount of this budget line, is supplied by donor funding. A donor might want to give to the SON but as unrestricted funds—not designated for anything in particular. The CNE can use these funds as she or he sees fit to benefit the SON.

This is a wonderful resource and can be used for anything from providing emergency funds to students in need to reimbursing the CNE for taking potential or active donors to lunch. Ask approximately how much there is in the discretionary fund and what, if any, are the restrictions.

The Budget "Ask"

The chief SON administrator may have the opportunity to ask for additional resources from the university or public university system. Nursing programs are often among the top money makers in the university because so many people want to become nurses or continue their nursing education. The SON administrator can make a viable case for expansion and thereby acquire additional funding for new facilities, equipment, and faculty.

This author was fortunate to work as dean with an amazing group of nursing deans who led the colleges of nursing within the same public university system. This group bears comment because they were incredibly collaborative and were as likely to share information with each other as other competitive deans might be to horde it. We met by phone regularly and in person as often as time and location allowed. Together, we developed talking points and white papers for regents and legislators. We recognized the shared need for additional resources to fund nursing education in our public system.

We were already familiar with the issues because they are the same across nursing education and particularly state-funded nursing education, among them the impending nursing and nurse faculty shortages due to the expected retirement of nurses and nurse educators over the next 5 to 10 years, the aging population, and the increase in the number of people living longer and with chronic illnesses. Together, we developed an aggregated "ask" or request for additional funding to expand our enrollments of bachelor of science in nursing (BSN) students. We also developed individual requests but collaborated with each other on writing introductions to these requests that reiterated the key issues facing nursing education and helped each other identify the primary resource needs and how to frame them.

Our requests included specific numbers of faculty and staff along with their salaries for each year of the biennial budget cycle. We included laboratory and simulation equipment and supplies and items specific to our units that would help us provide nursing education to more students.

Some asked for new facilities. Others did not need new facilities but needed additional simulators. The number of students by which we each hoped to expand varied depending on our plan and how much we could get for a finite increase in funding.

We approached our university chancellors and asked them to advocate for us with the university system. We gave them our aggregated and individual requests and successfully enlisted their support. This collaborative effort was very successful and is a perfect example of strength in numbers and of nurses at our best—working together to achieve a common goal.

Asking the Right Questions

If you are applying for an administrative role in a SON, know the questions to ask about the budget before accepting the position. It is unlikely that you will be given budget details until you are a finalist for the position and possibly not until you are offered the position. However, you should be able to glean the general amount budgeted to the SON as a total or parsed into tuition and state subsidy, program revenue, and revenue from auxiliary or other sources. For how much will you be responsible? What type of budget model is used from the system to the university? The university to the SON? Within the SON? What resources do you have to help you? Is there an SON budget analyst? Does the university financial services office provide mentoring and assistance? How knowledgeable or involved is the provost in the budget process for the SON? What is the president's background with regard to finance?

Do some research online and learn what the status of public funding is for higher education in the state. Do the governor and legislature support the public system and value higher education? Is there a tuition freeze and, if so, how long has it been going on? Have there been consistent budget cuts year after year? When did faculty last receive merit raises? What is university morale like related to budget? Spend significant time researching how the state views the university and whether there has been controversy related to financial (or other) matters. *The Chronicle for Higher Education* is one excellent and trusted resource to consider when researching these questions.

Salaries and some other budget information are publicly available. Take some time to explore and get a sense of how these salaries compare nationally. When did SON faculty and staff last get raises? The American Association of Colleges of Nursing (AACN) publishes faculty and administrator salaries for SON annually. How do the faculty and administrator salaries measure up?

As with so many other aspects of public university life, try to get a sense of the role of shared governance in budget decisions within the university system, university, and SON. How comfortable are SON faculty with their knowledge of and input in the budget?

■ THE FOR-PROFIT UNIVERSITY PERSPECTIVE

More often than not, organizations with a for-profit tax status are viewed as being focused on profit only. This is not true. Cowling and Groenwald (2017) assert that one should not a judge a nursing program by its tax status and they are absolutely correct. Programs should be judged on quality and selected on the basis of how well the program's mission, vision, structures, processes, and outcomes align with personal values and needs. Schools in the for-profit sector do run educational systems as businesses and, like all businesses, are concerned about the bottom line. But they are savvy enough to understand that you get a strong bottom line by providing quality and, make no mistake, regardless of tax status, when it comes to the budget, all schools and colleges are interested in profit. Therefore, appropriate allocation and utilization of resources is central to all leaderships positions, especially in the for-profit sector where performance appraisals and subsequent rewards (large bonuses and stock options) are based on both effectiveness and efficiency.

It is interesting to note that even though the dean or director is held accountable for managing the budget, he or she may not be involved in the budget development process. In some cases, the nurse leader may be able to request equipment or personnel during the budgeting process, but has no input in the decision-making process, where requests are evaluated and prioritized within and across departments. The role of the nurse leader will vary depending on the size, organizational structure, and, in some cases, state laws and regulations. Some smaller programs that are owned by families or individuals may not have a budget per se. I have worked in organizations in which there were no constraints on spending and items, such as paper, printing, postage, and lab supplies, were not even tracked at the department level. I got whatever I asked for as long as I justified the need. Although this seems like a desirable situation, it was also challenging. I had no constraints, but I also had no voice in how money got spent, how faculty were paid, and so forth. Involvement in the budget is a board of nursing requirement in most states, so although I could claim I had strong financial support, I was hard pressed to affirm that I participated in budget decisions. Unlike "mom and pop" schools, larger programs, especially those in which the nurse leader oversees operations and academics, will expect the nurse leader to be very involved with both setting and controlling the budget.

Setting the budget involves a series of conversations with department heads who are asked to project income from enrollment (admission and retention) and to project expenses, including fixed expenses, labor costs, staff development, capital expenditures, and costs of instruction such as testing and software licensing. If income is predicted to be strong based on market demand and historical data, the leader can plan to spend more money on staff development and recognition programs. On the other hand, if there is concern that income will fall below expectations, the nurse leader will not only have to cut back on staff programs but will likely have to cut back on staff as most budget overages or shortfalls are driven by labor costs. One aspect of managing the budget that is quite different in the for-profit sector is the level of involvement in admissions. The dean or director is expected not only to support admissions activities, but also to monitor enrollment on a weekly basis. In organizations in which the nurse leaders oversee operations and academics, there is likely to be tension between getting the numbers required to meet the budget and the quality required to matriculate students who will be successful on the NCLEX®. Nurse leaders in these organizations will be expected to have ready knowledge of not just admissions, but number of inquiries, how many inquiries led to applications, and how many of those converted to students who started the program. Some boards of nursing ask for these data annually so they can understand supply and demand within the state. Nurse leaders at for-profit schools are on intimate terms with these data and understand the "funnel" (how many applications it takes to create one enrolled student) well, as they are expected to meet targets.

Contrary to public opinion, admission representatives do not have or operate on a quota system. Nor do they receive compensation for enrolling a set number of students. This is against federal regulations. Admission targets are established for a campus based on income needs and all employees, (staff and faculty) are expected to help meet these targets. In the for-profit sector, variances to the budget are reviewed monthly so that course corrections can be made. In some organizations, these are high-level reviews and department heads are not involved, leaving control in the hands of the dean or director. I would advise involving department heads and, when it makes sense, team members in conversations about variance. Department heads make better budget decisions when they understand the impact of their spending decisions on their own department and other departments. When the team collaborates on spending decisions, funds can be moved and repurposed in a way that strengthens and invigorates the entire team as they work toward common goals.

As mentioned earlier, most boards of nursing and certainly the major nursing accrediting bodies require that the nursing program director be involved in some way in the budget process, even if it is only making capital requests or having input into the personnel budget. This fact can be used to leverage a stronger role in the budgetary process. Even the most reluctant administrations will have to demonstrate that the nursing leadership has some level of involvement in the budgeting process and that there is ongoing financial support for the department when the program sends in its initial self-study as well as its ongoing regulatory reviews. The nurse leader would be wise to get the regulations in front of the executive leadership well in advance of any board-required activity. I can remember an instance at a program early in my career when I asked the executive leadership to address capital expenditures in preparation for a visit from the board of nursing and the owner looked at the chief financial officer and said something like, "We probably should have a capital budget." I realized on that day that I had not asked nearly enough questions about the budget and my role in developing it during my hiring interviews or orientation to the role. If you are new to the sector, thinking about taking a leadership role in the sector, or opening a new school in the sector, I cannot overemphasize the importance of understanding the philosophy behind spending, and its relationship to recruitment of students, staff, and faculty, and how much you actually influence any of the decisions made.

In the for-profit world, you need to understand different types of budgets and budget cycles as well as how to read financial documents. You will be expected to forecast and control the budget, taking into account capital expenditures, building and equipment depreciation, staff and faculty salaries, and other items that contribute to the costs of instruction. Some terms to become familiar with and understand include *operating income (OI) percentage, average credit hours (ACHs) per student,* and *instructional cost per course (ICPC)*. You will not need to calculate these but you will be asked to defend them and take corrective action when they are below target. In almost all cases, the biggest impact on OI is labor in general, and adjunct salaries in particular. Controlling this expense through careful scheduling is key to managing the budget. ACH is another key area to manage especially if admissions or retention numbers are lagging behind those forecasted. Exploring why students are not taking the desired number of credits often reveals problems with advising, curricular structures (e.g., prerequisites), course scheduling, and faculty.

All institutions that are publicly traded must follow a set of generally accepted accounting principles known as *GAAP*. State and private institutions do not have to present their financial statements using GAAP, but according to the Government Accounting Standards Board, all 50 state governments do follow GAAP rules and guidelines. Adhering to these guidelines ensures accuracy, uniformity, and consistency in the way that financial statements are created and presented. In general, all financial statements should be objective, verifiable, and comparable. The most commonly used accounting principles are listed in Table 8.2. Understanding these principles helps you understand the financial documents you will be asked to work with. The school will provide a list of accounting codes called *general ledger codes (GLCs)* to help you identify the "pockets" that revenues and expenses flow into and out of.

Table 8.2 Commonly Used Accounting Principles

Principle	Definition
Going concern	Assumes that an organization will continue into the future
Monetary	Assumes the dollar is the unit of currency and that $1 spent in 1970 is equal to $1 spent in 2017
Cost	Refers to the amount spent at the time the item was obtained; there is no adjustment for inflation
Revenue	Refers to the practice of recording revenues as soon as they are earned as opposed to when they are paid
Matching	Requires organizations to match expenses with revenue; for example, salaries are entered when they are earned, not when they were paid
Conservatism	When faced with two alternatives for posting information, accountants are expected to choose the method that shows the least amount of net income to make the most conservative estimate
Full disclosure	Requires organizations to provide notes to help auditors or reviewers to understand accounting practices and decisions
Time period	Assumes that transactions occur over specific time frames that can be identified
Materiality	Allows the accountant to make decisions about how to account for an item using his or her professional judgement

Generally, the only revenue source is tuition. Expenses include fixed operating costs, such as rent, software licenses, and so forth, and variable expenses, such as faculty pay, student events, travel, development, community relations, library acquisitions, teaching materials, printing, office supplies, and so on. Colleges that have many campuses may "charge" each campus with a graduation fee so that the expense is shared across the system. Others may allow individual campuses to create their own graduation experience in keeping with what is available in the budget.

The GLCs help you plan and track these expenditures. Some programs may link team building and development and put it all in one GLC, some programs may put all travel together, whereas others will put travel for conferences in with conference and workshops. There is no right or wrong way to catalogue, organize, or track spending. At the end of the day, income needs to exceed expenditures. The nurse leader must use the assigned ledger codes to determine which ones are driving the bottom line. Is it a lack of income or excessive expenditures for adjunct faculty? Do you need to focus your efforts on advertising and, if so, which kind (print ads, radio spots, buses)? Or do you need to decrease spending? The executive will look to you for answers.

One difference between for-profits and not-for-profits is the profit margin expected. Most not-for-profits run on very slim profit margins less than 5%, whereas for-profit programs strive to be in the 15% to 20% margin. This makes sense when you consider there are shareholders to be paid and private owners are expecting to earn income from the business. Remember that multistate campuses must support centralized administrative services that have no direct tuition income stream. This profit margin becomes difficult for some individuals when they discover the "markup" that gets passed on to the student. Items, such as lab kits, may cost the student two or three times what they actually cost the program to purchase them. There are a number of valid reasons for this, but if this is a concern for you, the for-profit sector may not be the right place for you. Certainly, you should question any charges that you do not understand or have a concern about, but remember you have to make money to stay in business. This is true of all programs: public, private, and for-profit. Nurses often struggle with the idea of healthcare and educational organizations "making money." Even in hospitals, nurses are reluctant to charge patients for items they believe should be given freely or at a cheaper cost. The nursing values underpinning this reluctance can be upheld when you consider your duty encompasses the responsibility to be a good steward of the school's resources, fiscal and otherwise. In recent years, some for-profit schools have changed their tax status from "for profit" to "for benefit." This identifies the school as having a public benefit and indicates that some portion of the profits are used in support of that benefit. Maryland was the first state to pass legislation allowing organizations to have this status but the majority of states have followed suit (Neubauer, 2016).

Another budgetary consideration that is somewhat different in the for-profit sector is the "production value" of any given course. Programs in all sectors set enrollment requirements for courses to be able to run. Some for-profit programs often take this further and look at the college or university as a whole and limit the number of total courses/course sections that can be offered on any given campus. This is done in an effort to create fewer classes with bigger numbers to increase efficiency. This way of thinking works well in manufacturing, but does not translate as well in the education industry. Students like options, flexibility with schedules, and small class sizes, which is at odds with the production model. Student dissatisfaction can lead to fewer enrollments and a decrease in net promoter scores (NPSs), which ultimately negatively impacts the budget. Budgeting is a delicate balance between competing priorities and understanding the budgetary basis for class offerings is essential when you are building a schedule, thinking about hiring adjunct faculty to staff classes and clinical practica and balancing that against doing what is necessary to increase enrollment through recruitment and retention.

Depending on the accreditor, some for-profits must report satisfactory retention and placement scores to maintain accreditation. This quest for the numbers can make it challenging to maintain a focus on quality. You as nurse leader or responsible faculty member should keep quality at the forefront. There may be significant pressure to admit, save, or readmit students who have little chance of success. You have to hold the line. Remember that you have an ethical responsibility to both society via the social policy statement (Fowler, 2015) and the student. Is it unethical to continue to take money if there is strong evidence that the student will not be successful? Some would say yes. Others argue that adults have the right to pursue a path even if advised against it. Given the scrutiny on for-profit education, I would encourage that the decision be made with the student's best interest (as opposed to the organization's) in mind.

Another practice that needs to be carefully watched is that of interrupting classes for operation teams to have access to students. Persons from student accounts, registrar, career services, and so forth often have trouble getting students to respond to their phone calls, emails, and texts and like to use the classroom as an access point. The natural separation of academics and operations in public and private not-for-profit schools prevents this practice from occurring. However, there is no separation between these arenas in the for-profits. They are typically colocated physically and meet regularly for "all-hands meetings." Financial support for student activities may come from operations and academics so there is shared budgeting. Faculty may be asked to engage in marketing and demonstrate outreach as part of their evaluative process. In some organizations, NCLEX pass rates are used as performance measures for both operations and academics. The point is, there is a strong sense of "we are in this together," which is fine, even desirable, but may lead to blurred lines of academic ownership, which is not. Learning time is precious and needs to be guarded.

Ultimately, as a leader in the for-profit system you are expected to be profitable by managing income (admissions, retention, number of credits taken per quarter), and expenditures (labor, student activities, professional development, fixed expenses). The challenge is to do this without sacrificing quality. Understanding your market, working closely with the admissions team, planning carefully weekly, and reviewing monthly variances to the plan are key to your success.

■ THE PRIVATE UNIVERSITY PERSPECTIVE

Many nursing leaders rise up from the ranks of working as nurses or advanced practice nurses, then into a faculty role, and then advancing to leadership positions within academe. These promotions and advancement are often driven by achieving advanced degrees, usually in nursing or a related field such as curriculum and instruction, administration, or some type of leadership. In most cases, advanced education is accompanied with growing experience as a nurse or nurse educator. Depending on the advanced-degree program, nursing leaders may rise to leadership positions without having any formal education or any experience in developing or managing a budget over time.

Some nursing leaders may have experience with managing or monitoring a budget for a nursing unit. However, such budgeting experience often lacks the complexity that managing a budget within an academic nursing unit can have. There are nuances within academe that are different than what one would encounter in a healthcare setting. Therefore, nursing leaders who either strive for leadership roles or are taking on their first academic leadership role should take it upon themselves to gain an understanding of the budgeting process, how to work with spreadsheets, and learn some basic elements of cost accounting. This could be done through formal education (classes within a masters in business administration or nursing administration program) or more informal means, such as webinars or continuing-education programs, that focus on budgeting and effective resource allocation. There are often programs offered through the AACN, the American Organization of Nurse Executives (AONE), or other professional organizations to assist the nurse leader to become more knowledgeable in the area of budgeting and cost accounting.

Most budgets are divided into operating and capital expenditures. Operating budgets include salaries and benefits, costs associated with keeping the buildings on campus open and running, "taxes" paid to the university for departments that are not revenue producers (human resources and the library as was discussed in the public university perspective), and other ongoing costs necessary to do business. Because the operating budget includes salaries and benefits, these are often more "protected" in private universities. That is, even though academic leaders will have access to the operating budget, this often will not be shared with faculty and staff. Thus, this portion of the budget tends to be less transparent and available only to a select few. Personnel costs alone account for a great majority of the operating budget and significant changes to the operating budget can occur with changes in health insurance costs and other benefits from year to year. Nursing academic leaders often have decision-making power about salary for new hires, and they must consider how such salaries will affect the operating budget. For example, if a faculty member making $60,000 a year resigns and an SON dean wants to hire a replacement for $80,000 per year, that $20,000 increase in salary, plus the increase in the cost of benefits, will have to be accounted for in some way from 1 year to the next.

Typically, benefits range from 30% to 40% of an employee's salary and also have a huge impact on the operating budget. In the example in the previous paragraph, the person making $60,000 with a 30% benefit allocation means that person's salary line accounts for $18,000 in benefits. A new hire at $80,000 would have a benefit package totaling approximately $24,000. So not only does the base salary impact the operating budget, the benefits package also can have a significant impact, because an employee's retirement contributions, life insurance premium, and other benefits are often based on the base salary. Thus, a higher base salary translates into a proportional increase in benefits.

Capital expenditures have to do with equipment and supplies, travel, and other expenses that are not related to personnel. Typically, there is a process in place for requesting new capital purchases from 1 year to the next, with approval granted based on the needs of all schools and other ancillary departments. A savvy academic leader will gain input from faculty and staff related to real and anticipated needs and will have a process in place to prioritize requests and eventual purchases from year to year. Equipment that will contribute to increased enrollment or greater student success often becomes a high priority within a school and within the university. Similarly, equipment that affects the entire university to improve processes or procedures is typically a high priority, such as a more reliable or efficient learning management system, student information management system, or website upgrade. Because data-driven decisions are expected in all facets of higher education, investing in a more efficient and effective student information management system can be a high priority for every academic and nonacademic unit across the university.

Nursing academic leaders should be astute in determining depreciation values and the timing for replacing instructional equipment. Most universities have a plan in place to refresh technology, as computers and associated technology have a definite period after which upgrades are necessary. But lab and simulation equipment similarly have "shelf lives" and nursing leaders must do their best to predict and plan accordingly to upgrade simulators and manikins that will eventually wear out, no matter how well they have been maintained and cared for during their use. Because simulation manikins can range from $50,000 to over $100,000, it is best to plan over time for their replacement rather than expecting to receive approval for a replacement if a manikin breaks or "dies" after a period of time.

There should be routine maintenance funds included in annual budgets for simulation equipment and other high-priced instructional aids. Routine maintenance can cost $10,000 or more for each simulation manikin and expecting to "find" that money each year somewhere in the budget is not prudent. Just like healthcare organizations, some schools may choose to rent equipment, such as intravenous (IV) pumps, used in the skills and simulation labs rather than purchasing it, to save that steep up-front cost. However, healthcare organizations can often recoup the equipment rental fees by passing such fees onto patients using the equipment. It gets more difficult to pass fees onto students, unless course or lab fees are added.

Course or lab fees are often added to account for high-cost equipment or services needed for student learning. For example, many SON will have fees attached to clinical courses to account for the smaller numbers of students in each clinical section (each with one clinical instructor as opposed to larger numbers of students in theory courses). Clinical courses may be taught by adjunct faculty who are clinical experts, and a clinical fee may support the cost of hiring these adjunct faculty. In an SON, there is often a person who coordinates clinical placements and a person who may be responsible for ensuring contracts or memoranda of understanding are in place so that students can complete clinical rotations in healthcare and community settings. Clinical contracts are often reviewed by a university or system attorney. Liability insurance is typically carried by the school to cover students in the clinical setting. All of these services and the personnel who oversee these aspects related to clinical practica are "nonrevenue producing." Typically, it is the clinical course fee that covers these associated costs. Some schools will include the fee for criminal background checks, immunizations, drug testing, and other clinical requirements as part of a fee; other schools will have students pay for such services on their own.

Skills courses can also have significant direct costs associated with them. For example, a skills course could cost as much as $350 to $500 per semester per student to cover the cost of sterile and nonsterile supplies (catheters, IV supplies, dressing materials, medications, etc.). Students can often react negatively if they have to "reuse" supplies, but the reality is that such supplies are simply too costly to use once and discard. Sometimes, the thriftiness of reusing supplies in the skills lab will help students to be thriftier in the clinical setting, where waste can be very costly to patients and the organization.

Sometimes technology fees are associated with certain programs or individual courses. The Neighborhood™ or iHuman™ are examples of online learning technologies that might be used in some courses as teaching and learning aids. There are several options by which to pay for these technologies: (a) the school could pay for each student use, and take it out of some budget line; (b) the students could go to the website and register and pay for the program individually to gain access; or (c) a course fee could be added that will help the school recoup or defray the costs of using the technology. SON often do not have budgetary resources to cover the costs of these teaching technologies, which can be quite substantial, without adding a course fee or having the students pay individually to the company. If students are expected to register and access technologies on their own, and pay the fee directly, this cannot be covered by financial aid. Sometimes, if there are many additional costs, in addition to tuition, students will complain they are being "nickel and dimed" frequently. If a course fee is added, students can use financial aid to cover the cost. Therefore, a course fee is often more desirable.

Nursing leaders should review course fees on an annual basis to ensure the fee is still necessary and relevant. Leaders need to ensure that the technology or service that the fee was supposed to "cover" is still being used, is still necessary, and is still a good value. For example, a new faculty member might be hired and assigned to teach a certain course. The new faculty member may not have any desire to use a type of technology that was previously used in the course and may remove its use from the syllabus. However, unless this change is communicated to the registrar or accounts payable or whatever department assigns course fees, that fee will likely remain part of the student's bill. Students may not be diligent in scrutinizing their bills and may be inadvertently charged for something that is not being used. Reappraising the value of services regularly is also wise. Just like cable television, when services are first added in a nursing program, lower prices are often quoted to lure in potential customers. These prices can rise over time. Other companies may provide similar services or even better services for a more competitive price. As noted earlier, if nursing leaders treat the school budget as if it were their own money, they are more likely to be more astute in monitoring and implementing the budget.

Universities will often have a class size that is a breakeven point. That is, tuition and fees from a specific number of enrolled students covers direct and indirect costs of that course. That breakeven point varies in undergraduate or graduate courses, as tuition in graduate programs is higher. Because of the cost of benefits, full-time faculty are more "costly" than are adjunct faculty, who do not have the associated indirect costs of benefits. Therefore, academic leaders may have to make choices about whether it might be more fiscally sound to use adjunct faculty to teach classes with lower enrollments over full-time faculty. Similarly, full-time faculty with more seniority and higher ranks are often paid significantly more than newly hired faculty and those with lower ranks. Although nursing leaders have to ensure that all faculty members are academically and experientially qualified to teach any course to which they are assigned, a financial consideration may also have to be made when making assignments. It may simply not be cost-effective to have a PhD-prepared full professor teaching a BSN-completion evidence-based practice course in which eight students are enrolled. It may be more financially frugal to hire an adjunct with the necessary credentials, who is paid on a per-credit basis, to teach that course with a small number of students. Nursing leaders must keep in mind that the goal for any school or any program is not to break even, but rather to make money, so important decisions related to the budget must be made continually.

Dual-credit courses, in which high school students take college courses for a significantly reduced tuition rate (sometimes as little as $25–$50/credit), can be quite costly to a university. However, the exact benefit of dual-credit courses is hard to quantify, especially in the short term. Exposing high school students to your university is an important marketing strategy in the hopes students will have a positive experience and choose to attend the university for their baccalaureate degree. So, nursing leaders have to decide whether the short-term loss is worth an eventual long-term gain. Keeping data related to the number of dual-credit course enrollees who apply and enroll in the university will help academic leaders decide whether the investment is worth it. Using such evidence to drive decisions could help to justify offering more dual-credit courses, or to eliminate them from your school.

In undergraduate and graduate programs, events, such as welcome ceremonies, nursing pinning ceremonies, or student success initiatives, may not have budget lines associated with them. Academic leaders either have to itemize costs associated with such events (food, travel, honoraria) and assign costs to those specific budget lines or work to establish a budget line for such events. Although these events can be costly to operate, they certainly do contribute to the esprit de corps that will increase satisfaction and goodwill toward the school or program. Happy students become happy alumni, who have great potential to support the program after graduation both financially or through other involvement with students or faculty.

Private universities can have more leeway in moving funds between budget lines or categories than public universities have. Rules that guide what funds can be spent in what manner in the public sector are not as prevalent in private universities. For example, in a private university, funds may be moved from an account to support instruction into a fund to support faculty travel, where such a move may not be possible in a public university, depending on where the public funding was generated. Tax dollars or certain allocations may be restricted to certain expenses. This was detailed earlier in the public-university perspective.

Even though private schools are exclusively supported by tuition and endowments, like public universities the actual budgeting process can be very different from university to university. Similarly, the amount of control the academic leader will have over the budget-allocation process can vary significantly from university to university. Those seeking a leadership position need to ask direct questions about the amount of control or involvement they will have in the budget process. As noted earlier, accreditation standards require that nursing leaders have input into the budgeting process and allocation of resources. How much control and how that control is exercised can vary considerably.

Even though funding for public and private universities comes from separate sources, nursing leaders at private universities must stay attuned to what is happening in public universities in the state. As noted in the public university perspective, tuition at state schools can be frozen, often for extended periods of time. If state schools have a tuition freeze, leaders at private universities must critically evaluate their tuition rates. If a private university would raise tuition during a time when state schools have frozen tuition, the cost gap between public and private universities becomes even greater than normal. Therefore, even though private universities are not funded in any way by state budgets, what happens in relation to funding at public universities and what priorities there are related to education in the state budget does have an indirect impact on private universities. Therefore, it is prudent for leaders within SON in private universities to watch closely what is happening among the public sector and anticipate and plan for changes.

REFERENCES

Cowling, R., & Groenwald, S. (2017). Don't judge a nursing college by how it files its tax return. *Journal of Nursing Education, 56*(5), 255–256.

Fethke, G. C., & Policano, A. J. (2012). *Public no more: A new path to excellence for America's public universities*. Stanford, CA: Stanford University Press.

Fowler, M. (2015). *Guide to nursing's social policy statement: Understanding the profession from social contract to social covenant*. Silver Spring, MD: American Nurses Association.

Johnson, W. R., & Turner, S. (2009). Faculty without students: Resource allocation in higher education. *Journal of Economic Perspectives, 23*(2), 169–189.

Neubauer, K. (2016) Benefit corporations: Providing a new shield for corporations with ideals beyond profits. *Journal of Business & Technology Law, 11*(1), 109–129.

CHAPTER 9

MEETING ACCREDITATION AND STATE STANDARDS, ADVOCATING FOR YOUR SON

All schools of nursing (SON) strive to become and remain accredited by one of the three organizations given this responsibility: the Accreditation Commission for Education in Nursing (ACEN), the National League for Nursing Commission on Nursing Education (CNEA), and the Commission on Collegiate Nursing Education (CCNE). The SON must also have board of nursing (BON) approval within its state. Each state has its own regulations and policies that guide nursing education and practice. Most regulations are similar across states, but it is helpful to understand the variations. For example, state BONs often vary on how and when they waive the requirement for a graduate degree in nursing for instructors and faculty. Be aware of the regional and national guidelines followed by your university. For example, universities and colleges in New England are subject to the regulations and policies of the New England Association of Schools and Colleges, whereas Midwestern schools are subject to the Higher Learning Commission (HLC). All accrediting bodies must comply with federal guidelines established by the U.S. Department of Education (DOE) National Advisory Committee on Institutional Quality and Integrity (NACIQI). In other words, NACIQI accredits the accreditors. The Council for Higher Education Accreditation

(CHEA) also promotes academic quality. CHEA is a national advocate and institutional voice for its 3,000 degree-granting colleges and universities as well as its 60 institutional and programmatic accrediting organizations. It is a good practice to know what is currently going on in terms of accreditation at the federal level as well as current policy issues impacting higher education in general. Such information is readily available on the CHEA website.

Gainful employment refers to the extent to which colleges and universities prepare their graduates for employment in "a recognized occupation" (studentaid.ed.gov/sa/about/data-center/school/ge). Gainful employment has significant implications for the for-profit sector and are discussed more fully in The For-Profit University Perspective section of this chapter.

■ THE PUBLIC UNIVERSITY PERSPECTIVE

SON within public institutions are required to be accredited by ACEN, CNEA, or CCNE. Some prefer to be accredited by more than one organization. To become accredited, SON must write a self-study according to guidelines prescribed by the accrediting body. There are standards dealing with curriculum, fiscal responsibility, student success and satisfaction, and outcomes that must be specifically addressed. Some SON hire a consultant who helps them write the self-study document. They may also conduct a mock site visit to help prepare the SON for the real visit.

The self-study document is challenging to write. This author recommends assigning the coordination of the self-study and the visit to someone who can devote the necessary time to it, preferably someone who has been directly and significantly involved in academic accreditation visits previously, and who is very well organized and can write well. The task definitely requires a coordinator; however, it is ideal if other members of the SON contribute to the document and to the visit. It can be extremely helpful to assign people who logically fit with one of the accreditation standards to gather the information and write portions of the standard. For example, faculty who have experience developing and evaluating curriculum should be assigned to assist with the standard pertaining to curriculum. Faculty who work with program outcomes should work on the standard that requires the SON to demonstrate student and faculty achievement and progress. A clear timeline and roster of whom is accountable for what specifically is worth its weight in gold. The coordinator gathers the information from others and inserts it in the self-study document, where appropriate. As the document begins to take shape, multiple readers from within the SON and the consultant (if you are lucky enough to afford one) should review it for clarity and comprehensiveness. Also, it is tempting to use acronyms and abbreviations that an outside reader might not understand. A glossary is helpful. Box 9.1 provides some tips for writing a good self-study document.

The accrediting body determines when the site visit will be and organizes a team of visitors whose expertise closely matches the content of the programs in your SON. For example, the SON may have a traditional bachelor of science in nursing program, a master of science in nursing specializing in the clinical nurse leader, and a doctorate of nursing practice specializing in the family nurse practitioner. The accrediting body will assemble a team that has expertise in each of these areas. Often the team consists of deans and directors who have experience as faculty and as administrators. It is a wonderful opportunity for the site visitors to visit various SON because the visits enable them to learn about other ways of educating nursing students and stimulate new ideas.

Accrediting agencies have seminars whereby deans, directors, or faculty can learn about the requirements and any changes that have occurred in accreditation expectations. It is wise to attend these approximately 1 year prior to the visit. Accrediting organizations are ready and willing to help by phone with any questions SON have.

Accreditation site visits are very stressful but employing systematic processes to prepare for and organize the visit can minimize last-minute stress. As with so many things, communication is key: Communicate with the lead site visitor about the team's preferences for organizing materials, communicate with faculty and staff throughout the preparation for the visit and development of the self-study, and communicate with university leadership to ensure they will be available and understand the importance of the visit.

Box 9.1 Tips on Writing a Self-Study

- Read the standards and requirements carefully
- Respond to what is being asked
- Use data and examples to illustrate points
- Start collecting data at the very beginning of the period being evaluated (usually 3 years); however, have processes in place all of the time for gathering and analyzing these data
- Have faculty collect student exemplars
- Collect alumni achievements, including awards, publications, promotions, and employment
- Collect faculty achievements, especially publications, presentations, grants, and awards.

The self-study should not be viewed merely as a necessary evil, but as a terrific learning experience. If done correctly, it sheds light on the strengths and weaknesses of the SON and requires in-depth analysis of what has not gone so well and what can be done better.

The self-study is submitted to the accreditor prior to the site visit so the visitors have sufficient time to review it prior to the visit. The visit typically occurs over a 2- to 2½-day period. At the conclusion of the visit, the team will inform the dean and the SON whether it has any concerns or recommendations for improvement; however, final word about accreditation approval occurs after several months. During that time, the accrediting organization may request more information or material to help inform its decision.

The Academic Nursing Administrator's Role in Accreditation and BON Standards

The academic nursing administrator is ultimately responsible and accountable for the success and viability of the SON. Before accepting the position, so he or she should learn about the past status of the SON. Has it always been accredited? If so, when was the first accreditation? By which organization? For how long? Which organization(s) accredit the SON currently? Were there any recommendations or concerns from the accrediting body during the last accreditation visit? If so, what were they and have they been corrected? When is the next accreditation visit? You do not want to work for an SON that is not accredited or is not planning to actively seek accreditation.

BON Statutes

When applying for a position in another state, find out whether it is a compact state and the requirements for licensure well in advance of your move (see Box 9.2). Some states require a lot of paperwork. As an administrator or as faculty, an awareness and understanding of your state's BON statutes can be very helpful as you hire faculty and educate students. If you are also engaging in your own clinical practice, understand the expectations within your state. If your school is in an area that borders other states and jurisdictions, faculty will have to hold a license in the state where the school is located. If faculty teach a clinical course in a bordering state, they will also have to be licensed in that state. Each state has a higher education commission that must be petitioned in order to have an educational presence within that state. Although this approval is a university- or college-wide concern, it may impact the nursing program if the program is operating clinical practica outside the state. Maryland, for example, does not allow bordering states to have an educational presence

Box 9.2 Sample of State Boards of Nursing Activities

- Approval for SON
- Licensure
- Examining councils
- Renewal of license
- Standards of practice
- Rules of conduct
- Certification of advanced nurse prescriber

SON, school of nursing.

without approval from the Maryland Higher Education Commission (MHEC), and does not allow outside nursing programs to establish clinicals within their state lines. On the other hand, Maryland's neighbor, the District of Columbia, does not have any such restrictions. It pays to check ahead of time.

Other Nursing Education Standards

As has been mentioned elsewhere in this book, the SON has its own standards, which are outlined in the student and faculty handbooks and in the SON bylaws. The university will also have a faculty constitution and bylaws. The university faculty senate is responsible for developing standards that pertain to faculty and it behooves administrators to understand these policies.

Advocating for Your SON

Deans and nursing academic leaders are often required or encouraged to meet with legislators or members of the Board of Trustees or Board of Regents to advocate for nursing issues. Public universities, in particular, pursue legislators to obtain funding and support for higher education. The nurse academic leader who seeks out and creates opportunities to rub elbows with legislators and regents can establish relationships and educate the people who decide on policy and funding.

It is helpful to reach out to legislative staff to invite legislators to tour your facility or to join the SON for a special event. Many of the faculty, staff, and students are likely to be constituents of the legislator so it behooves the legislator to be seen as supportive of the university and the SON. Encourage the university chancellor/president and provost to invite you to lunches or leadership meetings when legislators or regents come to campus.

If the SON gains approval to offer a new program, moves into a new facility, develops a simulation center, acquires an endowed professorship, celebrates an anniversary, or does something otherwise noteworthy, work with the university public relations and marketing staff to get on the news and in the newspapers. Encourage the public relations staff to contact you when there is a healthcare issue in the news and to utilize you and your faculty as healthcare experts. This will increase the visibility of the SON and the university.

Invite regents and legislators to see what you are doing and share in your accomplishments. As discussed in Chapter 4, create an annual event, such as a fund-raiser for student scholarships, which will bring the community and legislators to your campus and increase the visibility of the SON.

Have a message that is always ready that you can deliver to the decision makers. Keep the message straightforward and consistent and make sure it is supported by data. Work with your public relations staff to craft a coherent and strong message. For example, SON in public universities often need additional monies and resources to expand. As the nurse academic leader, work with your faculty, public relations staff, and advancement officer to craft a message that clearly explains that more nurses are needed to care for the citizens of your state in the future, especially as the baby boomers age and live longer. Use data from the American Association of Colleges of Nursing (AACN), the National League for Nursing (NLN), and the American Nurses Association (ANA) that show national nursing trends.

Then use data from your state organizations to show the current and impending shortage of nurses and nurse educators in the state and predictions about future healthcare needs to illustrate the need for new nurses. Conclude with three to five "asks." For example, ask for more money to educate nurses to become nursing faculty, more money to hire doctorally prepared nurse faculty to teach students, and more space/a new facility to house classrooms for expanded numbers of students. The message should be confined to one page.

Whenever you are in contact with a legislator or regent, convey the message and leave behind a hard copy. Email this individual a few days later and thank him or her for taking the time to speak with you and be sure to reiterate your message.

Another excellent way to get through to legislators, especially, is through state dean and director organizations. These organizations might have different names but often include nurse educators and/or administrators from both public and private universities within the state. They may also include nursing programs for an associate degree, diploma, or licensed practical nurse, as well as university programs. This is an excellent way fornursing programs to work together toward common goals. For example, members of this organization might agree that no SON in the state will pay preceptors so that they do not add extra competition between SON that can afford to pay and those that cannot. The organization might agree to develop and utilize a database for all clinical placements so that each SON has an equal opportunity of placing its students in locations within the state. It might also work to develop an orientation for new preceptors.

A major strength of organzations is seen with regard to working on state issues. There is strength in numbers. If a statewide organization of nurse educators brings a proposal to the legislature, it is more likely to get heard and addressed than if SON work independently.

Nurse academic leaders who sit on executive boards and are active in state and national nursing and healthcare organizations have opportunities to get to know the "movers and shakers" within the state. This increases their visibility and credibility and the likelihood that their voices will be heard. Encourage your faculty to obtain positions on boards throughout the state. This involvement will also give you a voice in influencing and making policy.

Be sure your provost and university chancellor/president are aware of your message and approve you sharing it. You do not want to be viewed as going around your administration and you want to be sure your message is consistent with the university's strategic plan and mission. Frequently, the university chancellor/president will want to initiate the contact with the legislator before you contact them. The same is likely to apply to the Board of Regents or Trustees. The provost is your boss (assuming you are the dean; the dean is your boss if you are a director) and you should not surprise your boss or put them in an uncomfortable position when they speak to regents or legislators.

Whenever possible, try to get involved in health policy issues on a national level. The AACN deans' conferences are helpful in this regard, especially because of the formal Capitol Hill visits deans make in state teams during the conference time. The national nursing organizations are excellent in providing synopses of issues that impact nurses and that nurses can influence. There are also regular calls from these organizations to nurse leaders to help develop or change policy. At a minimum, attend conferences and read the literature to keep current with what is happening in nursing and healthcare.

■ THE FOR-PROFIT UNIVERSITY PERSPECTIVE

When it comes to accreditations and regulations, the nursing programs in the for-profit sector must meet the same standards as those in other sectors. The state BONs and the accrediting arms of the AACN and

NLN do not alter the standards or benchmarks based on program type. This is the great unifying factor for programs and the hallmark of quality that should provide the detractors of for-profit programs with sufficient evidence that (a) our graduates are on par with other programs providing high-quality healthcare and (b) for-profit programs are providing a valuable service to the communities they serve.

There is as much variance within a sector as there is among sectors. In the area of compliance, the variation is not in whether the standards are being met, as not meeting standards results in sanctions up to and including closure of the program. The variance lies in the level of accreditation (regional vs. national), how the data are collected and presented, who has the responsibility for this effort, and the resources available for this purpose.

The majority of for-profit schools started out as career colleges, which explains why many of them are still accredited at the national level. Many career colleges began to move away from offering vocational certifications to providing higher degrees. For some, this change in educational scope created a desire to move to regional accreditation. Regional accreditation makes it easier for students to continue their education at mainstream schools and in some ways makes programmatic accreditation easier as the standards and outcomes for nursing are much more in alignment with those of regional associations and commissions. National accreditation focuses on retention and career-related outcomes such as placement, whereas regional accreditation focuses on quality of faculty and student learning outcomes. National-level accreditors, just like regional accreditors, must be approved to operate by the NACIQI in the DOE. In 2016, for-profit schools in general and one of their major accreditors, the Accrediting Commission of Independent Colleges and Schools (ACICS), came under increased federal scrutiny. This scrutiny led to decertification of ACICS (an action still being contested in the courts at this writing), leaving more than 200 schools and thousands of students in jeopardy of losing federal aid and hundreds of faculty in fear of losing their jobs. Nursing programs that find themselves in a situation in which the university has lost accreditation must contact the BON to ensure that graduates will be eligible to sit for licensing exams.

A major driver of the heightened scrutiny mentioned in the previous discussion is the issue of gainful employment. The remarkable growth of the for-profit sector spurred consumer advocates and educators to examine outcomes of the sector. Researchers began to suggest that graduates from the for-profit sector had more difficulty finding employment and higher debt and default rates than graduates from programs serving the same demographic populations, especially community colleges (Cellini & Turner, 2016). In 2009, the DOE began exploring the role of career colleges and ways to impact student outcomes. In 2012, the judicial system found that the DOE did have authority to regulate these schools and in 2014 the gainful employment regulations were finalized. Beginning in 2015, schools must provide an accounting of students' debt-to-earnings ratios. To receive financial aid, graduates must be employed in a recognized occupation that provides enough income to meet the following criteria:

- Student loan payment is less than 20% of discretionary income
- Student loan payment does not exceed 8% of annual earnings

According to a DOE press release (2017), over 90% of the schools that failed to meet the gainful-employment rule were in the for-profit sector. Certainly, the nursing graduates in these programs are meeting the gainful-employment standard, but the data are reported in the aggregate for the college or university as a whole. Therefore, as either leader or faculty member you should be aware of the college or university's performance in this area as it impacts financial aid and military benefits for all students. Career Education Colleges and Universities (CECU), the trade organization that represents career colleges, has lobbied strongly against the gainful- employment rule on the basis that it unfairly targets the for-profit sector. Other than public or not-for-profit certificate programs, the gainful-employment rule is only applied to for-profit programs. CECU maintains that all those in higher education should be held accountable. How many philosophy or creative writing majors, for example, could meet the gainful-employment rule? Not many. Fair or not, the gainful-employment rule is in place and you need to be aware of the placement rate of the nursing graduates and how the college or university is doing vis-à-vis the regulation. Failure of the school to meet the standards can have disastrous results for all involved. Losing federal financial aid, which is the primary source of income for for-profit schools, could lead to budget cuts and ultimately closure.

National Versus Regional Accreditation

A list of organizations approved by the DOE to accredit schools at both the national and regional level excerpted from the DOE website is provided in Table 9.1. You will note that regional accreditors, unlike national accreditors, limit their scope to colleges and universities that offer degrees within specific states and territories (regions). National accreditors cover schools across the country but limit their scope to the types of programs offered.

Accreditation on every level is a factor to consider before accepting employment or promotion, as you will have a significant role in collecting the data and writing the self-studies associated with the accreditation process. Many for-profit nursing programs are new start-ups, meaning

Table 9.1 Organizations Providing National-Level and Regional-Level Accreditations

National-Level Accreditation	
Accreditor (Year Opened/Year of Next Review)	**Scope of Recognition**
ACCSC (1967/2021)	Accredits postsecondary, non-degree-granting institutions and degree-granting institutions in the United States, including those granting associate, baccalaureate, and master's degrees, that are predominantly organized to educate students for occupational, trade, and technical careers, and including institutions that offer programs via distance education.
ACCET (1978/2018)	Accredits institutions of higher education throughout the United States that offer continuing education and vocational programs that confer certificates or occupational associate degrees, including those programs offered via distance education.
COE (1969/2021)	Accredits and preaccredits ("Candidacy Status") postsecondary occupational education institutions throughout the United States that offer non degree and applied associate degree programs in specific career and technical education fields, including institutions that offer programs via distance education.
DEAC (1959/2017)	Accredits postsecondary institutions in the United States that offer degree and/or nondegree programs primarily by the distance or correspondence education method up to and including the professional doctoral degree, including those institutions that are specifically certified by the agency as accredited for Title IV purposes.

(continued)

Table 9.1 Organizations Providing National-Level and Regional-Level Accreditations (*continued*)

National-Level Accreditation	
Accreditor (Year Opened/Year of Next Review)	**Scope of Recognition**
MSCSS (2004/2017)	Accredits institutions with postsecondary, non–degree-granting career and technology programs in Delaware, Maryland, New Jersey, New York, Pennsylvania, the Commonwealth of Puerto Rico, the District of Columbia, and the U.S. Virgin Islands to include the accreditation of postsecondary, non–degree-granting institutions that offer all or part of their educational programs via distance education modalities.
TRACS	Accredits and preaccredits ("Candidate" status) Christian postsecondary institutions in the United States that offer certificates, diplomas, and associate, baccalaureate, and graduate degrees, including institutions that offer distance education.
Regional-Level Accreditation	
MSCHE (1952/2017)	Accredits and preaccredits ("Candidacy status") institutions of higher education in Delaware, the District of Columbia, Maryland, New Jersey, New York, Pennsylvania, Puerto Rico, and the U.S. Virgin Islands, including distance and correspondence education programs offered at those institutions.
NEASC, Commission on Institutions of Higher Education (1952/2017)	Accredits and preaccredits ("Candidacy status") institutions of higher education in Connecticut, Maine, Massachusetts, New Hampshire, Rhode Island, and Vermont that award bachelor's, master's, and/or doctoral degrees and associate degree–granting institutions

(continued)

Table 9.1   Organizations Providing National-Level and Regional-Level
Accreditations (*continued*)

Regional-Level Accreditation	
Accreditor (Year Opened/Year of Next Review)	**Scope of Recognition**
	in those states that include degrees in liberal arts or general studies among their offerings, including the accreditation of programs offered via distance education within these institutions.
North Central Association of Colleges and Schools, the HLC (1952/2017)	Accreditation and preaccredits ("Candidate for Accreditation") degree-granting institutions of higher education in Arizona, Arkansas, Colorado, Illinois, Indiana, Iowa, Kansas, Michigan, Minnesota, Missouri, Nebraska, New Mexico, North Dakota, Ohio, Oklahoma, South Dakota, West Virginia, Wisconsin, and Wyoming, including the tribal institutions and the accreditation of programs offered via distance education and correspondence education within these institutions.
NCCU (1952/2018)	The accreditation and preaccreditation ("Candidacy status") of postsecondary degree-granting educational institutions in Alaska, Idaho, Montana, Nevada, Oregon, Utah, and Washington, and the accreditation of programs offered via distance education within these institutions
SACSCOC (1954/2017)	Accredits and preaccredits ("Candidate for Accreditation") degree-granting institutions of higher education in Alabama, Florida, Georgia, Kentucky, Louisiana, Mississippi, North Carolina, South Carolina, Tennessee, Texas, and Virginia, including the accreditation of programs offered via distance and correspondence education within these institutions.

(continued)

Table 9.1 Organizations Providing National-Level and Regional-Level Accreditations (*continued*)

Regional-Level Accreditation	
Accreditor (Year Opened/Year of Next Review)	**Scope of Recognition**
Western Association of Schools and Colleges: junior division focuses on community and other colleges with a primarily prebaccalaureate mission (1952/2017); senior division focuses on senior colleges	Accredits and preaccredits ("Candidate for Accreditation") community and other colleges located in California, Hawaii, the U.S. territories of Guam and American Samoa, the Republic of Palau, the Federated States of Micronesia, the Commonwealth of the Northern Mariana Islands, and the Republic of the Marshall Islands, which offer certificates, associate degrees, and the first baccalaureate degree by means of a substantive change review offered by institutions that are already accredited by the agency, and such programs offered via distance education and correspondence education at these colleges.

ACCET, Accrediting Council for Continuing Education and Training; ACCSC, Accrediting Commission of Career Schools and Colleges; COE, Council on Occupational Education; DEAC, Distance Education Accrediting Commission; HLC, Higher Learning Commission; MSCHE, Middle States Commission on Higher Education; MSCSS, Middle States Commission on Secondary Schools; NCCU, Northwest Commission on Colleges and Universities; NEASC, New England Association of Schools and Colleges; SACSCOC, Southern Association of Colleges and Schools, Commission on Colleges; TRACS, Transnational Association of Christian Colleges and Schools, Accreditation Commission.

they have not graduated enough students to have full board approval (this usually requires having at least 1 year's worth of pass rates) or programmatic accreditation from the NLN or AACN, or they have only received approval for a shortened amount of time, for example, 5 rather than 10 years. Some state BONs will provide longer approval periods if the school has ACEN or CCNE accreditation. Multisite programs are likely to have a team that interacts with accrediting agencies and BONs as well as either assisting with or writing self-study documents, but small programs will look to the dean/director and faculty to accomplish those tasks. Keep in mind that some accreditors require a "midcycle report," which also involves submission of an updated self-study. Make no mistake, whether initial or ongoing accreditation, the process is an enormous undertaking. Some schools have invited the state board to renew approval status (note state boards approve, national agencies accredit) sooner than required in order to synchronize approval and accreditation cycles. Because state boards and national accreditors require much of the same data, it reduces the burden by addressing all standards in the same time frame once a decade rather than going through the process repeatedly every 3 to 5 years.

Advocating for Your SON

Leaders and faculty in the for-profit sector often find themselves in a position of defending the sector and confuse that activity with advocacy for their program. Although you should understand the mission and vision of the sector as a whole, the best way to create a positive image in any sector is to promote quality programs within the sector and then work with those programs to bring about positive change. The first step is knowing your program strengths and the myriad ways it serves the communities of interest. The next, and more difficult step is getting a seat at the table. Investigate opportunities to work on committees and task forces within local, state, and national nursing and healthcare groups and organizations. Attend national nursing meetings and encourage faculty to present posters and papers. This helps to establish your program and you as being on par with public and private programs and their leaders. Being "part of the club" strengthens your voice and broadens your area of influence. Contact local NLN and ANA chapters, check out the health department website, and see what the current initiatives are. Explore opportunities to join city and county boards that work within the healthcare arena or have a related purpose. An opportunity that many for-profit schools take advantage of is joining the chamber of commerce. The chamber provides a wide variety of networking events that lead to opportunities for clinical sites and educational partnerships. If you are working in a program that is publicly traded, any public activity or messaging needs to be approved before proceeding, but in every situation remember that you are the face of the program and need to be circumspect in your language, behaviors, and associations.

Another avenue for advocacy is to seek and apply for voluntary recognition programs. For example, the NLN offers schools the opportunity to be recognized as a center of excellence. Chamberlain University, a multisite for-profit nursing program, was recognized in 2016 as a center of excellence in the area of promoting the pedagogical expertise of faculty. Recognitions such as these open dialogue across sectors and support claims that quality programs can exist and thrive in the for-profit sector.

■ THE PRIVATE UNIVERSITY PERSPECTIVE

Accreditation Standards

Because SON in private universities are accredited by the same organizations as public universities (ACEN, CNEA, or CCNE), what was written in the public-university perspective applies equally to private universities. One aspect that is slightly different is that private universities do not have to publicly disclose faculty and administrators' salaries, so that information can be withheld from self-study documents and other reports to accreditors. Salaries at private universities are often lower than their public and for-profit counterparts, which provides some rationale for withholding such information. However, this author believes that reporting those salaries to accreditors is actually beneficial, considering the information can provide more accurate comparison data to other SON, which can help academic administrators to make a case for ensuring that compensation packages within the SON are equitable compared to other organizations. Accreditors' recommendations can prove to be very strong and compelling with administrative leaders. For example, an accrediting team could recommend that salaries at a private school are not competitive with other like organizations, which could lead to the inability to recruit and retain qualified faculty either currently or in the future. Such a recommendation could have a profound impact on administrative leaders to support salary increases. As noted earlier, maintaining accreditation is a top priority for SON leaders and university administrators alike.

The maximum CCNE accreditation is for 10 years. Of course, there are many changes that typically occur within schools and their programs during a 10-year accreditation period. Substantive changes in programs or in program outcomes need to be reported to accrediting bodies according to their guidelines in between self-studies or accreditation visits. CCNE has specific guidelines detailing what substantive changes need to be reported. These include a major curriculum change, change in administrative leadership for the program, and a significant change in human or financial resources to support the program(s), among others. Specific requirements and a template for recording substantive change can be found on the CCNE website. There are specific timelines in which these substantive changes can be reported.

The maximum ACEN accreditation is 8 years. ACEN has requirements comparable to those outlined for CCNE for reporting both planned and unplanned substantive changes. Examples of planned substantive changes include organizational structure changes within the SON, implementation of distance learning within a program, and additions of new programs or new credentials. Unplanned substantive changes include changes in state BON approval or declines in program outcomes such as NCLEX® pass rates of the SON's graduates, among others. The specific guidelines can be found on their website. Leaders within SON need to be keenly aware of the accreditation requirements and stay abreast of any new and ongoing developments. Failure to comply with notification requirements, even if inadvertent, could lead to negative consequences for the program. Academic leaders need to be attuned to the specific requirements of their accrediting organization as well as the timing in which to report any changes or to submit required documents in order to remain compliant.

As was noted earlier in the public university perspective, writing self-study reports can be a daunting task. However, organized academic leaders will use principles of continuous improvement and keep ongoing records of relevant information that will be necessary to compile the self-study report, whenever it is due. If deans, directors, and faculty are keenly aware of the accreditation standards and the key elements for each standard, information to support how the school and the program are meeting those standards can be continually saved throughout the accreditation period. This provides specific, relevant, and ongoing examples over time that accreditors look for in a self-study.

If a school's programs are accredited for 10 years through CCNE, school leaders will have to write a continuous-improvement progress report (CIPR) to be submitted at the 5-year midpoint. Self-study and CIPR reports typically focus on the prior 3 years of data immediately before the submission of the CIPR or the accreditation self-study. At this author's university, files named for each standard and key element are saved on a shared drive. Any time an example to support how the school and its programs meet the key element, it is saved on that shared drive in the appropriate file. When it comes time to write the next self-study or CIPR document, much of the necessary information will be readily available.

Similar record keeping can be done with meeting minutes, in which actions are taken and information about those actions are documented. Anyone who has poured over months' or years' worth of meeting minutes looking for when a change was made or a policy was voted upon and implemented can attest to the tedious and frustrating nature of such a search. However, keeping a master list of each committee's major motions, resolutions, and policy changes on one spreadsheet that includes the date that items were discussed and passed can save a tremendous amount of time and effort, especially as it relates to compiling the self-study or CIPR document. Such a list can serve as a table of contents that can direct leaders to the correct meeting minutes in which to review the more complete account or action. Meticulous record keeping, with the accreditation standards in mind, can make formulating a self-study a much easier task as all the data that was saved in real time will be readily available. This is much more efficient than trying to recollect and reconstruct documents directly before the self-study is due to support how the SON met the standards during the past 3 years.

Sometimes academic leaders will volunteer to be an accreditation site visitor or will encourage one of their faculty members to do so. This is one way to gain added comfort with accreditation standards, site-visit procedures, and to see how other schools are meeting accreditation criteria. This is an important professional service that should be encouraged by university and SON leaders.

Besides being meticulous about maintaining program accreditation through the appropriate nursing organization, academic leaders also need to consider regional accreditation guidelines or standards that apply to the university, such as those of the HLC. Typically, a university will have an internal liaison or resource person who is the go-to regarding HLC standards and is responsible for conveying information or updates to the rest of the university and to assist academic leaders to meet current or updated standards. Sometimes this person might be a faculty member or academic administrator who serves as an HLC site visitor; sometimes it is a person who is accountable for reading and staying up-to-date on any changes. HLC also has a designated liaison to universities, a key resource for questions and to provide information about standards. Be aware of what programs or changes need to be reviewed and approved by HLC prior to implementation. For example, a new doctoral offering would need HLC approval, including a site visit prior to implementation, but a new master's certificate may not need such approval, especially if students in the certificate program would not qualify to receive federal loans. In fall 2017, the HLC is implementing new standards for faculty qualifications for teaching. Accredited schools will have to review faculty teaching loads and compare those to faculty's academic and experiential expertise to ensure that the new standards set by HLC are met.

Dealing With State BONs

State BONs all have individual standards as well as ongoing reporting requirements; some states have much more stringent requirements than others. Most state boards put the greatest emphasis on prelicensure programs and those graduate programs that lead to certification as APRNs. All state BONs have a consistent goal to protect the public in ensuring that licensed nurses (practical and registered) and APRNs have met the minimum standards necessary to carry out their scopes of practice. That is the reason for state boards having the greatest interest and oversight in prelicensure and APRN programs.

As noted earlier in this chapter as well as in Chapter 7, when an academic program has students who are completing clinical rotations in another state, leaders must determine what approvals are necessary from that state BON prior to students entering the clinical rotation. It can take as long as 9 to 12 months to achieve state BON approval for programs to offer clinical rotations and some states will not grant approval for out-of-state students to complete clinical rotations in their state. This author has extensive experience seeking multiple state BON approvals for a prelicensure second-degree distance education program. The process involved in working with each state board, with its unique and individualized requirements for program application and ongoing reporting, was extremely labor intensive and daunting at times. Some state boards meet less frequently than others, which can delay action related to an issue or request. Typically, deadlines are in place to submit materials in order to get on a state board meeting agenda, and those deadlines can be difficult to uncover. Even if on an agenda, some state boards will finish a meeting once the allotted time has elapsed, even if the agenda was not complete. This can leave a request or application to be put off for another month or 2. If an academic leader has traveled to appear before the state board, a second or even third trip may be necessary (see Chappy, Stewart, & Hansen, 2010, for a more detailed account of dealing with state BONs and recommendations). Many states have cut funding to BONs making it difficult to find a person who staffs the office with whom one can speak on the phone. Thus, getting information from a person can be difficult, leaving the website as the main means for which to obtain information about board policies and practices. Some state board websites are much easier to navigate than others.

At this author's university, for each state in which we have nurse practitioner (NP) students, we had to go through an application and/or notification process to ensure that our students could complete clinical rotations in their home states. State BONs are typically not concerned about nurse educator students' clinical rotations because these students are already licensed nurses and are not completing clinical to lead to a new caregiving certification; thus, no oversight on the part of the state BON is typically necessary. Overall, dealing with compact states if the SON's state is part of the compact is typically easier regarding compliance with requirements, but it varies considerably from state to state. Some states require hefty annual application fees that make it cost prohibitive if there are only a small number of students from that area. Some states have extensive application and/or reporting requirements that make it cost prohibitive and time intensive for an SON to maintain all the necessary requirements. As noted earlier, some states do not allow out-of-state students to complete clinical rotations. Based on all of this information, universities and SON often develop a comprehensive list of states in which they are approved and from where they can accept or not accept students. Often one person may have to be dedicated to reviewing and documenting state BON requirements in each state in which students are completing clinical practica to ensure a change or update is not missed. Noncompliance with a standard or not meeting a deadline, even if inadvertent, could result in a fine, withdrawal of approval, or students being unable to begin or complete their clinical rotations.

This author is dean of an SON at a university that has two residential campuses, one in Wisconsin and one in Michigan. In 2015, we began investigating the possibilities of offering the traditional nursing program, which was already accredited in Wisconsin, at our Michigan campus. This would mean crossing state lines with BONs in two states. Crossing state lines is common with for-profit universities, but is less common for public and private universities. We began by searching the Michigan state BON website and discovered that a member of that board happened to live in the city in which our Michigan campus is located. We contacted her with the intent of asking questions and seeking advice regarding barriers and facilitators we would encounter if we moved forward to seek approval of a new prelicensure program in Michigan. This person provided much insight about the Michigan board's actions and past decisions that assisted in our planning.

We conducted market research (using an outside company to eliminate bias) that proved to be important in showing the Michigan board members that the current and future demand for nurses was strong, even though there were several baccalaureate nursing programs already established in the immediate geographic area in which our campus is located. We obtained information from the Michigan state BON website regarding application and approval processes. We learned that a significant determinant for approval would be the availability of clinical sites. Our next steps were to set up meetings with nursing and administrative leaders at area healthcare organizations and community agencies to seek support for our intended program.

During our visits with nursing and administrative leaders at the healthcare organizations, we were informed of some challenges that we may encounter, specifically bottlenecks that can occur with some specialty clinicals and the lack of adequate space even for programs already in existence in the area. Leaders encouraged us to structure our program in such a way that specialty clinicals like obstetrics and mental health be offered during "off times" such as the summer months or winter breaks. We were informed that inpatient pediatric placements would be especially difficult to secure, which led us to investigate opportunities to place our students in summer camps and other community settings where they could successfully meet the pediatric clinical course objectives. We found that public health settings, which cannot typically accommodate as many students as acute care agencies, were already at capacity with students from existing programs. This information led us to explore offering community clinical rotations in underserved areas and as part of global experiences.

Even though we were offering the same curriculum in Michigan as we were in Wisconsin, and were meeting the same course objectives, we did not have to offer the courses in exactly the same sequence. Knowing the potential challenges we would face, we could order the courses in such a way as to maximize the available clinical opportunities, and to be creative in exploring and designing new opportunities. Having a sound plan that we tailored as a result of the information we received from the board and area healthcare leaders provided a strong foundation for our initial application to the Michigan state BON.

Another key decision that supported our successful initiation of this program was hiring a campus dean for nursing for the Michigan campus. She was a key facilitator in ensuring we got all necessary board documents submitted by the deadlines, she arranged for the initial state board site visit, and had community connections to secure additional support for clinical rotations. Having boots on the ground with a person familiar with local culture and resources was critical in moving this initiative forward in a timely manner.

As we were planning the program, another early conversation occurred with contacts at CCNE, our accrediting body. We learned that because our program was already accredited in Wisconsin, we would need to submit a substantive change notification 90 days before or after we initiated the program in Michigan. Our story may not be unique, but it represents the persistence and diligence necessary in dealing with state BONs when initiating new programs or revising existing ones. Academic leaders need to understand the necessary processes with licensing, accrediting, and certifying bodies, as well as with state BONs.

Advocating for Your School

Advocating for your school with legislators and other key stakeholders is similar to that reported in the public university perspective. Private schools are not affected by state budgetary considerations as are the public universities becauseprivate schools are funded by students' tuition and endowments and they do not receive state aid. However, all schools, whether public, private, or for-profit, are affected by similar faculty shortages, student loan concerns, and having limited resources to offer nursing programs. Therefore, any efforts to work collaboratively with public and for-profit universities to advocate for legislation that improves nursing education or contributes in some way to improving the profession of nursing in the region and in the state can be noteworthy and mutually beneficial.

Federal policies and initiatives affect all SON equally. For example, Title VIII funding to support nursing education and research affects all SON in the form of grant and research dollars available for which all SON can compete. As noted in the public-university perspective, concerted efforts to support initiatives involving academic leaders at all SON that affect all schools within the state will result in a stronger voice and a more powerful message to legislators.

REFERENCES

Cellini, S. R., & Turner, T. (2016). *Gainfully employed? Assessing the employment and earning of for profit college students using administrative data* (NBER working paper No. 22287). Cambridge, MA: National Bureau of Economic Research. Retrieved from http://www.nber.org/papers/w22287

Chappy, S., Stewart, S., & Hansen, T. (2010). Eliminate border wars: A call for action. *Nursing Education Perspectives*, *31*, 392–394. Retrieved from http://search.proquest.com.cuw.ezproxy.switchinc.org/docview/853717751?accountid=10249

U.S. Department of Education. (2017, January 9). Press call to announce for debt-to-earnings rates for gainful employment career training programs. Retrieved from https://www2.ed.gov/news/av/audio/2017/01092017.pdf

CHAPTER 10

EXPLORING INNOVATIVE IDEAS AND STUDY ABROAD

Academe is looking for innovative academic leaders—people who are not only open to new ideas but have a storehouse of them. When you apply for a leadership role, especially as chief nurse executive, you will inevitably be asked to describe your vision. How can one truly espouse a realistic vision when she or he has not yet experienced the culture or life of the school of nursing (SON)? Yet, this is the inevitable question and must be satisfactorily answered if you have any hope of being offered the position. What the faculty and staff of the SON may really want to hear is that innovation is possible and that the prospective leader has new and brilliant ideas that will lead the SON into the future. Although the prospective leader's vision may not end up being the hired leader's ultimate vision, neither should be pulled out of thin air. Both the prospective and final visions should be based on close study of the characteristics and goals of the faculty and staff, the environment in which the SON resides, and the trends occurring in that environment.

Prospective faculty are not typically asked about their vision for the school but are often asked about their experiences innovating in the classroom, their use of technology, and the techniques they use to engage students—who are harder to engage than ever before. Study abroad (SA) is included in this chapter because although not innovative in and of itself, it presents opportunities to broaden students' minds and to expose them to new ideas and people from different cultures.

■ THE PUBLIC UNIVERSITY PERSPECTIVE

Common themes throughout this book from the public university are the decline in the perceived value of public higher education and the scarcity of resources. From the public university perspective, innovation is not simply the buzzword of the day, but a necessity. People must constantly do more with less, which inevitably requires new ways of seeing and doing things. It is something of a contradiction to expect innovation without making additional resources available to support new ideas. That is not to say that there are not ways to be innovative and creative for free or at low cost.

Professional development programs can be useful in many ways to the new and experienced academic leader. Some are more helpful than others. One of the programs this author attended was the outstanding American Association of Colleges of Nursing (AACN)–Wharton Executive Leadership Program. I highly recommend it to other nursing academic leaders. Some of the pearls gleaned from the program are included in this chapter. At the conclusion of this chapter, other sources that may be useful to the reader are listed.

The academic leader may start the job excited and enthusiastic and full of new ideas, but consider these thoughts from Fethke and Policano (2012):

> Visionary . . . leaders do not receive the bonuses expected in corporate life; rather, they face strife, contentious and sometimes hostile meetings, and little hope of achieving real change. A sobering reality is that the most likely reward for anyone who proposes strategic, innovative change that involves trade-offs is a short tenure in office. Paradoxically, achievement of broad consensus may be most effective for sustaining leadership even if everyone is marching in the wrong direction. (p. 177)

Faculty may say that they want change—cultural change, curricular change, structural change—but whether they are willing to participate in making change happen is another thing altogether. The process of effecting change may be difficult at times, but the end result can be very worthwhile. Convincing faculty of this is not always easy. Administrators take a risk when they suggest change. I experienced faculty dissension when, in response to severe budget cuts, I asked faculty to look at their workloads. Workload is one of the sacrosanct areas for faculty, especially in public universities in which faculty governance plays a huge role. However, workload is directly related to the financial resources of the SON. Other areas in which I tried to innovate involved looking at research and scholarship differently. Both areas—workload and scholarship—had not been touched for many years so it was challenging to help faculty see that the current and projected public university environment not only required change but could be the impetus for innovation.

Breaking established patterns of thinking and helping people to be open minded and to not feel threatened by change and innovation are challenging, especially among senior faculty who are often entrenched in old ways of doing things. Senior faculty may contend that an excellent board pass rate justifies keeping things the way they are and there is no cause to embrace new strategies. Joe Perfetti of the Wharton Executive Program (personal communication, August 8, 2016) described other pitfalls that can impede innovation:

- Identifying the wrong problem
- Aborting too quickly
- Stopping (with the first good idea)
- Failing to identify a "potential antagonist"
- Obeying rules (that do not exist)

Innovation is often born of the need to solve a problem. What actually is the problem and what should be done about it? It is worth spending ample time to study the problem and analyze its etiology. As we learned at the Wharton School, people are most likely to ask, "What's in it for me?"

Stopping the process of change too quickly and before people get into the groove of sharing new ways to problem solve and innovate can end or stall the entire process. Rules exist to be obeyed and nurses are the kings and queens of rule following. However, testing a relatively low-risk idea and preparing to respond to those who might be likely to oppose it are often worth the effort and the risk. Joe Perfetti described Prather's (2010) list of nine workplace dimensions that support innovation:

- Challenge and involvement
- Freedom
- Idea time
- Idea support
- Positive agitation and conflict
- Debate
- Playfulness and humor
- Trust and openness
- Risk-taking

I have found it worthwhile to keep these dimensions in mind. However, some items on the list present challenges in SON. "Idea time" must somehow be found in and among classes, clinical practica, faculty practice, simulations, research, and scholarship. Faculty often feel overwhelmed as it is. Nurses are not natural risk-takers. We are trained to be scientific and systematic. Although we must be adaptable to new environments, risk-taking jeopardizes patient safety and patient safety underlies our core. Nursing faculty must be encouraged to take risks in their thinking.

Although nurses are not reluctant to debate, challenge, or become involved, junior faculty, who by virtue of their relative youth and inexperience might be more open to new ideas, may feel intimidated by senior faculty, who will ultimately recommend their promotion and tenure. Junior faculty are frequently stifled, whether intentionally or unintentionally, from saying what they think. This is why the nursing administrator should try to create and maintain an environment in which challenges to the current ways of thinking and doing are invited and welcomed and not viewed as threatening. Senior faculty may not view themselves as impediments to progress and many are not; however, the nursing administrator should try to enlist the support of senior faculty if the environment is to adapt to change. "Positive agitation and conflict" are good as long as they remain positive and do not become an attack on the people who are trying to bring about change. The Wharton School recommends using the STAR model:

- Be specific (S)
- Take small steps (T)
- Alter the environment (to move people in a direction) (A)
- Be a realistic optimist (R)

Taking risks and shifting resources to allow for innovation is a new way of thinking for many faculty. Wharton also recommends "rapid experiments" that can be accomplished on a small scale. They call these "test and learn" opportunities. The desired outcome is to learn from the trial, not to measure its success or failure. Testing is the reward. Remaining vigilant and teaching faculty and staff to remain vigilant for new ideas creates an open environment. Everyone is exposed to a potential new idea every day. An environment that welcomes new ideas will encourage employees to take the next step of vocalizing and sharing these ideas. Being able to "pivot" when something is not working is also a key. Although aborting too early can jeopardize potentially great changes, knowing when to give up on a great idea is also important.

Innovative thinking is at the core of strategic planning. Where does the SON want to be in 3 years? In 5 years? Involving everyone, including clerical staff and students, in strategic planning immediately sets up an environment in which new ideas are expected and welcomed. Doing so sets the tone that the SON belongs to everyone, that everyone has a say in where it is headed, and that everyone is responsible for what happens next. Joe Perfetti of the Wharton School says that there must be "a concise and clearly communicated description of where the organization will be such that everyone clearly understands the ultimate objective" (personal communication, August 8, 2016).

On becoming dean at one SON, I became aware that strategic planning had previously only involved tenured faculty and the dean. The plan was skeletal and underdeveloped. I held a 2-day retreat focused on strategic planning. I brought in an expert from the College of Business at my university. Brainstorming led to specific goals and strategic initiatives. Faculty and staff divided themselves into groups based on their interest in these initiatives and then "elected" champions or facilitators to lead each group. Each group met monthly to work on specific action steps against a timeline they created. As dean, I met with the facilitators every month to hear about their progress and to share my activities so my efforts could inform their work and vice versa. Over time, faculty and staff realized that not everything could be accomplished in 3 years and began to prioritize their action steps. Some people attended all of the meetings and were heavily involved in strategic planning, whereas others seemed less interested. In any case, everyone had the opportunity to participate and have a say in where the SON was headed. Buller (2014) claims that strategic planning does not work and can actually impede transformative change. Rather, scenario planning or a strategic compass is preferable.

Kathy Pearson, also of the Wharton School, suggests that the key barriers to strategic agility include a strong set of assumptions, not recognizing what we do not know, only seeking information that confirms what we believe, and resistance to change (personal communication, August 10, 2016). She contends that we should not just seek to change things when they are broken, but we must always be thinking of the future. To plan for the future, she recommends identifying the uncertainties (trends), tracking the key uncertainties, and taking action around the key uncertainties, such as conducting tests and learning experiments. In nursing, we know that people are aging, there are more people living with chronic illness, that global infection is a growing concern, and that we are increasingly using technology to assess and deliver healthcare. These are predictable. According to Dr. Pearson, we need to focus on what is not predictable or the "unknown unknown." Nurse administrators need to be adept at scanning the environment for trends from outside the United States and outside healthcare, not just from the usual sources.

Dr. Pearson also advises that leaders make sure that everyone understands the intent of change and why something is being changed or a change is proposed. Clarity and prioritization matter more than the volume of communication that takes place. The people who will actually be implementing the change can also put up the most barriers against the change. They should be involved early and often.

Strategic agility, according to Dr. Pearson, requires being able to make a decision even when you do not know what will happen. Overanalyzing before making a decision can lead to not making a decision. I have known several nurse leaders who overanalyzed and who have missed unique and promising opportunities. Red teaming (Hoffman, 2017), an approach that has its origins in the military, involves carefully selecting people who are intentional devil's advocates so the leader is exposed to why the project will not work as well as how it can work.

Study Abroad

International study and experiences are wonderful ways to expose students to other cultures and new ideas. Faculty who accompany students are likely to also learn a great deal that can inform their teaching and scholarly work. An international trip is a wonderful way for students to apply clinical learning in an environment that may not have the abundance of resources we are accustomed to in the United States. Students may take courses alongside students from the country they are visiting. This also provides perspective on how other nations provide education. Students frequently return with a completely new outlook that ultimately makes them better nurses. Faculty often return tired but reenergized and excited to share their experiences.

Students sometimes have opportunities for internships in other parts of the United States. Although English is more likely to be predominant, these opportunities may also expose students to areas in which poverty and access to healthcare shed light on the healthcare disparities that remain in our own country. I once had a graduate student question why I taught so many hands-on techniques in the graduate health assessment course instead of teaching students to rely on imaging studies to identify disease. The class took place at a very well-respected research university. I explained that MRI machines and other equipment that can diagnose disease are not readily available everywhere and that clinicians must be able to rely on their own skills to diagnose and treat. Living in the modern age, students may not realize that not everyone can afford or access sophisticated diagnostic testing techniques or treatments.

There are many variations in SA opportunities, from very short trips in which nursing students can work on specific projects in underserved areas in other countries to semester- or year-long programs and internships. Students (and faculty) should understand that although Americans tend to be casual in our interactions with others, other cultures may be more formal in both dress and interaction. On an SA trip to Peru with nursing students, I noted that while in clinical, the Peruvian students were very neat with their hair pinned up and with little to no makeup. They interacted with and addressed faculty in a more formal way than I was used to.

Not only is it preferable that nursing students represent the United States and the university well, but they should be mindful that they represent the American nursing profession. Other cultures tend to admire how far and how fast our profession has grown. Not all countries (few in fact) have advanced practice nurses and not all have the same degree of autonomy we have worked so hard to achieve. Representing nursing professionalism, but also showing respect for the nursing profession in other countries, is incumbent on students and faculty alike. A nursing faculty member once told me she danced on the bar with her students when they were on SA trips. Not only is the use of alcohol among nursing students while abroad questionable, but even faculty who have good relationships with their students must model professionalism and cultural sensitivity.

An international studies coordinator who coordinates trips can be helpful to ensure that faculty and staff follow guidelines. Most public universities have university departments for international education. Find out exactly what they do and what the SON is expected to do to organize and supervise SA. Making assumptions about these functions will only lead to trouble and may jeopardize the trip.

■ THE FOR-PROFIT UNIVERSITY PERSPECTIVE

Innovation is an arena where for-profit programs excel. Although for-profit education has existed since ancient times (Cannella & Finkelstein, 2008) and flourished in the form of trade schools in the late 1800s, it did not really capture the attention of academe until Richard Sperling started the University of Phoenix in 1976, lending a new "legitimacy" to the sector (Ruch, 2001) and paving the way for large corporations with a lot of capital to open multicampus colleges and universities. There are many such corporations but three that are publicly traded and quite well known include the Apollo Group, which is the parent company of the University of Phoenix; Adtalem Global Education, which is the parent company of Chamberlain College of Nursing; and Strayer Education Inc. These large corporations have the agility, technologies, and financial support to bring new ideas to practice quickly and efficiently. Ruch (2001) describes these corporations as both leaning and cutting edge. The actual number of for-profit schools that offer nursing is unknown as players continually move in and out of the market. Some well-known programs that are not publicly traded include ECPI University, Rasmussen College, Stratford University, and South University. What all of these schools have in common is the ability to operate in a "lean" fashion while bringing advanced technologies to their programs. They tend to be early adopters of technology and most have exquisitely appointed simulation centers and learning support labs that incorporate the latest advances in education such as virtual reality platforms to enhance learning. Although not the first to offer courses outside the "brick-and-mortar" classroom, for-profits were the first to promote online learning as a replacement for entire curricula.

The for-profits very successfully answered the market demand for "distance education" and now remote learning is a preferred way of matriculating for thousands of students, most of whom are not geographically distant, but unable to attend structured synchronous classes on campus. Hybrid or blended courses have also been developed in response to market demand for students who have limited time but enjoy some face-to-face contact or support.

For-profits also offer a great deal of flexibility in course offerings and scheduling. I had the opportunity earlier in my career to open a nursing program and actually polled the students as to the days and times they would like to attend class. That group chose to have all didactic classes on 1 day to free up clinical days that would work around their lives. Because schedules are created "just in time," for-profits can move classes around to fit student preferences up to and including the first week of class. Most for-profits run 8- to 10-week terms. This allows for early and timely evaluation of courses and clinical sites that inform and influence scheduling and hiring and allows for increased responsiveness to student needs. The downside to just-in-time scheduling is the shifting of clinical sites and faculty that it requires. It is imperative to honor commitments to all of our partners. Last-minute changes can create a negative image with faculty and clinical partners. These changes need to be carefully constructed so that the same faculty member or agency is not repeatedly impacted. Sometimes running a clinical practicum with less-than-desirable enrollment is preferable if cancelling damages your relationship. Short-term wins should not trump long-term gains. Act in the moment with the long-term view in mind. Most adjuncts understand that they will occasionally lose a course to low enrollment, but when it happens repeatedly you are likely to lose the adjunct.

Another benefit accorded to the larger multicampus programs is the opportunity to pilot a new technology or innovation on a single campus, work out the kinks, and implement it across all campuses rapidly. Because most colleges and universities have very flat structures, decisions can be made in one session and implemented in the next. Of course, this can also be a challenge as frequent, rapid change can be a dissatisfier for both faculty and students. This is especially true when there has been insufficient time to "roll out" the change. The changes that seem to occur most often and present the biggest challenges are changes to the learning management system (LMS; Blackboard, Moodle, e-College, Canvas, etc.). Very often updates to the LMS are done without warning and sometimes complete changes from one platform to another are done with very little time to get fully oriented to the new platform. Because for-profits are able to move quickly, organizational leaders often do so without fully understanding the time it takes to accept and incorporate change at the local level. Although change is constant for everyone, constant change can be demoralizing and as a campus or program leader you need to embrace change while managing and messaging it carefully. Students in particular are affected by change. It creates anxiety and stress in an already stress-filled experience. Communication is key to change management. A phrase used often in the for-profit sector is "seven ways seven times," which means you have to overcommunicate to deliver the message and you have to find a medium that resonates with your students. Remember that the for-profit student profile is typically female, working, between the ages of 30 and 50, and from a minority or underserved population. Communication methods need to include texting, email, print, video, face-to-face, and social media formats.

Although there is a great deal of focus on the academic experience and innovation in teaching, the for-profit schools are always looking for innovative ways to enhance the student experience as a whole. One of the ways that for-profit programs differentiate themselves is through what has been termed "wrap-around services." This means that a relationship is forged with each student at the time of admission that continues through graduation. One example of this is the Chamberlain Care Model, which provides early assessments of risk that lead to customized support plans, coaching, and workshops that address life challenges as well as academics (Cowling & Groenwald, 2017).

Study Abroad

International education is available at most for-profit colleges and universities. In fact, many have campuses established in countries around the world. The difficulty for students is financing the extra expense and managing the time away from home (remember the demographics) and other life commitments. Students have to pay for the course credit as well as the cost of travel. Students who have been able to participate in a learning-abroad experience report it as "life changing" and well worth the expense. Global education and student testimonials related to these experiences are strong marketing tools that help to differentiate your program and tend be well supported at the highest levels of leadership.

Untapped opportunities for the same type of experience lie in courses that occur in underserved U.S. populations and locations such as Native American reservations, disaster stricken areas, and pockets of extreme poverty in rural areas. Given the agility and just-in-time nature of the for-profit sector, these courses could be developed and implemented rapidly at relatively low cost for the student. As a leader in a for-profit organization, you will able to identify and operationalize these types of opportunities much faster than in the traditional educational sector, sometimes within a single academic calendar year.

■ THE PRIVATE UNIVERSITY PERSPECTIVE

At a recent faculty meeting, during a curriculum and assessment review, one faculty member shared that at a recent conference a keynote speaker often remarked, "Remember when we used to do XYZ " or, "Remember when ABC was part of the curriculum?" The faculty member brought this up because XYZ and ABC were still parts of our curriculum and were part of the discussion that day. Many times, those who are noninnovators will say, "If it ain't broke, don't fix it." Faculty may believe a curriculum is working just fine if NCLEX® pass rates are high, but they may not be looking at a 60% attrition rate within the program, which is simply not acceptable by accreditation standards and by ethical standards. It would be easy to weed out all weaker students and boast a high NCLEX pass rate. An academic leader takes all outcome information into account. Although NCLEX pass rates are critical, academic leaders will tell you they are merely one measure of a successful program.

Successful academic leaders will continually fix things and innovate when things are not broken. Everything will break eventually without preventive maintenance. When academic leaders only make changes when things break (NCLEX scores fall, attrition increases, admission numbers plummet), this leads to a reactionary mentality; those changes can often be haphazard, knee-jerk responses to an immediate problem. The time to make change and to innovate is when things are going well; when details of change or a new process can be well thought out and implemented in a way that is not reactionary to a problem but rather is a forward- thinking, evidence-based decision to improve.

Some would argue that many nursing curricula still look like they did 50 years ago "because it works." Course names reflect fundamentals, health assessment, skills, medical/surgical nursing, obstetrics, pediatrics, research, community health, policy and politics, and leadership and management, which are not unlike the course names this author enrolled in during her undergraduate nursing education in the 1970s.

Certainly content has been updated, but the foundational concepts remain quite similar. In the 1970s, the term *informatics* was not in existence. Using information meant referencing published sources to justify a nursing action or support a stance on an issue. Interprofessional education was just getting noticed, but more in relation to working with other disciplines to care for patients. Research classes focused more on doing research than on applying research to influence practice. Since the 1970s, how we get and use information has changed exponentially.

In the 1970s, we located journal articles, which were available as print copies on the library shelves or by request through an interlibrary loan that took 2 to 3 weeks to receive by mail, by using the big red Cumulative Index to Nusing and Allied Health Literature (CINAHL) books that were updated and published several times a year. This was quite different from online search functions available through the library with millions of full-text articles immediately available to students within minutes. Today's students have information at their fingertips at every point of education and patient care, yet we often ask them to put their phones and other devices away during class. Many healthcare organizations do not allow students to access material on their phones while in clinical. Do such policies really make the best use of the information that is so readily available to help them make evidence-based decisions?

Healthcare has also changed exponentially and continues to change on a daily basis. If you went to an orthopedic surgeon, and the surgeon told you the hip replacement you were to undergo would be done exactly like it was in the 1970s or even in the early 2000s, you likely would seek another opinion (or at least you *should* seek another opinion). In academe, if nursing leaders and faculty are not continually updating and upgrading curricula; revising processes, marketing plans, and strategic directions; and reviewing feedback from internal and external stakeholders and developing strategies to act upon that feedback, they will lag behind and be left in the dust by those who are doing so. Nursing students simply cannot be prepared to care for the patients of today; they must be prepared to care for patients of the future who are receiving healthcare in places and in ways that have not even been invented yet. Who would have thought 50 years ago that there would be clinics in retail outlets, or we would be using computers, phones, and other handheld devices to assess, diagnose, and treat patients. So what does the future hold for healthcare delivery? That is a great question upon which to speculate.

It is so true today that nursing curricula are packed with content. Noninnovators believe that the only way students will learn something is if it was "said in class." How many times have you heard something like, "I don't know why they all got that wrong on the test; I said it in class." Today's students are digital natives, which makes them unlike their faculty counterparts in most cases. Nursing leaders and their faculty must develop ways to help students learn to find information rather than making sure that content in courses gives them the information that faculty believe students will need "when they get into practice."

So how do you encourage innovation and creative thinking? One way is making sure there is some time for thinking. A second necessity is a "playground" that is ripe for thought and idea sharing. When this author was attempting to balance school, work, and a home life, one very respected professor noted that I needed to take time to think . . . to let all the readings and doctoral work sink in. I worked diligently to schedule "downtime," which may have been something as simple as turning off the radio while driving when I was alone in the car to give me time to think about my scholarly work, the things I was reading, and my program of research. It helped tremendously. I found myself carrying a small notebook (these were the days before cell phones) and I jotted notes to myself to include on papers, to bring up in class, or even to think about in more detail later. I found myself writing down a lot of questions, which stimulated broader and deeper thinking. I got "there," according to this professor, who truly instilled in me the need to get off the hamster wheel that is our day-to-day responsibilities and have time to get lost in thought; to develop the "what if . . .," "why can't we . . .," and "why don't we try . . . " ideas.

As noted in the public university perspective, academic leaders recognize that faculty are all extremely busy with teaching, scholarship, and service requirements. It takes time to innovate and innovation takes thinking. Do faculty have enough time to think and have "idea time"? Do faculty need help to slow down and not get so caught up on the treadmill completing routine tasks of updating syllabi, revising course materials, revising exams, collecting data for research endeavors, publishing, and participating in meetings, among other expectations for the faculty role? Academic leaders need to be savvy at planning and implementing activities, retreats, or downtime that promote camaraderie and allow time for faculty to clear their heads and think. This is time that is very well spent.

Academic leaders also have to work to establish a clear picture and understanding among faculty that innovation and change may not always be successful. Anticipated outcomes may not come to fruition when new ideas are implemented. Faculty and staff must understand that lack of success of a new initiative is a viable option. New ideas may not work as planned, and that should never be reflected as a failure. If there is any evidence of a punitive culture, change will never be supported. Academic leaders can typically identify those faculty members willing to try new ideas; those are individuals who have confidence in themselves and their work. Those individuals need to be allies and their successes should be highlighted; their "failures" should be addressed as a learning opportunity and a chance to do a root cause analysis. Sometimes, when there is not a tenure system in place, or when senior faculty are not the ones recommending promotion, junior faculty will be less afraid to innovate and try new things. Lack of success on one endeavor is not seen as a deterrent to future success.

Innovative cultures should not imply that "anything goes." Savvy nursing leaders and faculty will take calculated chances and will not do anything that disregards accreditation standards, board of nursing rules, or the best interests of students and other stakeholders. However, there may only be a slight difference between a culture of innovation and one of the "Wild West." Some risks are worth taking; you may have to ask for forgiveness later if they do not work out, but other risks need to go through the proper channels to avoid potential ethical or legal ramifications.

Private universities tend to have fewer levels of approval and tend to be able to be more responsive or receptive to change and innovation than their public-university counterparts. Some believe it can be difficult to be innovative and separate your SON from other SON, especially considering that almost all programs must meet accreditation standards through one of the nursing accrediting bodies (Accreditation Commission for Education in Nursing [ACEN], the National League for Nursing Commission on Nursing Education [CNEA], or Commission on Collegiate Nursing Education [CCNE]) and universities must meet similar regional or national accreditation standards. This in and of itself causes some similarities in curriculum, policies for admission, retention and progression, and assessment and evaluation procedures. All nursing programs seek to have graduates with high pass rates on the NCLEX or advanced nursing certification exams. However, nursing leaders at private organizations must develop ways that differentiate their programs from others, especially considering the higher cost of tuition. Having innovative approaches to teaching and learning are ways that private organizations can distinguish themselves. Some examples might include developing innovative interprofessional clinical opportunities like those at this author's SON, where nursing students participate with students from social work, physical therapy, occupational therapy, and pharmacy in experiences such as a working in methadone clinic, participating in smoking-cessation classes, drug court, and in-home safety screening for participants in a home meal program.

The advancement of online education was detailed in the for-profit university section of this chapter. Many private universities have similarly embraced distance learning from its inception. In fact, at this author's university, early adopters of online education were actually given the freedom to become a "separate" department within the university so they were free to move at a faster pace in adopting online technologies and teaching methodologies than the rest of the university was willing to do. Those early innovators did not want progress slowed.

As a result of this freedom, the university has become a known leader in distance education among private schools. This "separateness" from the rest of the university is now being eliminated as the rest of the university has "caught up" in using online education and distance learning technologies to deliver courses and programs. That "division" that was created so the innovative faculty would not be held back is no longer necessary as the rest of the university is on board with paving the future in developing and implementing creative and innovative course delivery options and teaching methodologies. Nursing leaders need to allow departments, divisions, or individual faculty to launch innovative ideas and creative methodologies on a small scale without having to get the entire school on board. Again, these small tests of change or offerings, as one nursing leader called a "school within a school" concept, can lead to a less-threatening environment for those who may be unwilling to take a leap into a new process or procedure until they can see results from a smaller pilot. What might be their initial no vote can be swayed to a yes vote using positive results from a pilot test. What might be their initial no vote may never have to be tallied if the pilot does not work and the idea is not advanced.

One of the greatest complaints heard from nursing faculty concerns their salaries being less than competitive, especially once immersed in academe and knowing all of the expectations that accompany the faculty role. This author uses innovation as part of annual evaluations. Faculty and administrators must define what they did different this year as compared to the past year. If they have nothing to report and they are doing everything the same, they know that means they did not meet my expectations. I ask them why I should authorize a salary increase or extra rewards if they are doing exactly the same things they did the year before; what warrants more pay for doing the same thing? At least this has prompted some of them to think about innovation, if only once a year. Other faculty bring a laundry list of what they tried in the past year and what they want to try in the future. With persistence, the entire faculty group, or a great number of them, can be moved to a culture of innovation.

Sometimes nursing leaders need to adjust assignments or teaching loads to accommodate change. For example, at this author's SON, the clinical paperwork assignments for the medical–surgical courses were very outdated, repetitious, and did not reflect current practice or current evidence-based recommendations. I had nudged faculty to make changes, but only minimal adjustments were made over a period of 2 years. Finally, the students became very vocal about not only the assignments and their perceived dissatisfaction with them, but also with the timing for due dates, timing of faculty feedback, and the impact that completing the very arduous clinical assignments was having on students' ability to study for, and focus on other coursework. I changed the course coordinator so that a new direction could be forged. Of course, I did this with no malice, but simply noted to the previous coordinator that I expected a new direction and after 2 years, I did not see meaningful results. Therefore, I appreciated her ongoing and continued input, but someone else would be leading the revisions. Changes like this also send a message to others that change is necessary in order to stay current, maintain a strong curriculum, and prepare students for the realities of current and future nursing practice.

During the clinical assignment debate, one faculty member noted that she refused to make changes during the semester, but would consider doing so next semester. That meant that students who had taken the initiative to speak up could not be affected by any improvements. Although it was a stretch, I likened this to the Tuskegee Syphilis Study, when no changes were made to the study protocol even though penicillin had been discovered to effectively treat syphilis. I encouraged that faculty member to not be afraid to "make things better" for students even if mid-semester. I would never increase rigor or add assignments in the middle of a semester, but I certainly advocate for making improvements at any point of time.

Nursing leaders need to learn to surround themselves with thinkers and doers, especially those who complement the leader's skills and abilities. This author is more of a "big thinker" and once an idea takes shape, I do not always see the best or most efficient way to implement that idea. I have learned to surround myself with people who are detail oriented and willing to weigh the pros and cons of operationalizing strategies. If I would surround myself with only other big thinkers and ignore those who can work out the details of how to get things done, I would be left with a lot of ideas, but little action. Sometimes, the detail-oriented people and big thinkers can drive each other crazy, but the smart ones know they have a very mutually beneficial symbiotic relationship in which success can only be accomplished when they work together as a team to come up with innovative ideas and then implement them in the best possible manner.

Innovation can be related to course offerings. Many traditional undergraduate nursing programs offer courses in a traditional format during the spring, fall, or summer semesters. But offering courses in 4-, 6-, 8-, 10- or 12-week formats rather than during a full semester could positively affect students' schedules. Innovation lies not only in content, but in method and timing of delivery as well. Innovative leaders know that every course does not need to be three credits, but having three one-credit courses, especially if those teaching the one-credit courses make it three credits worth of work, can be detrimental to student scheduling. Offering courses between semesters during an interim term or even over spring break can be positively received.

There has been much debate over massive open online courses (MOOCs) and their value in higher education. This is not the forum to discuss the pros and cons of MOOCs. However, creating MOOCs to expose high school students to your school, to the profession of nursing, or to some type of nursing content (math for meds, in-home caregiving, navigating the healthcare system, etc.) can be an excellent marketing tool and pique the interest of those who enroll in the MOOC. Many schools are investigating policies and procedures for transferring or accepting credit for prior learning related to work completed in MOOCs. MOOCs seem to be here to stay, so investigating their positive contribution to higher education is worthwhile.

A summary of advice regarding innovation is included in Box 10.1.

Study Abroad

Private universities often use SA options to further support and extend their mission, which could include service work in the United States and global locations, as has been described in the public university perspective. In addition, global locations can provide excellent clinical opportunities for students in all specialties. In this competitive nursing education environment, where there is strong competition for clinical sites, offering global clinical experiences provides the cultural exposure in a diverse healthcare setting as well as providing care to people who have different health practices than students are used to seeing.

The benefits of global experiences for students and faculty alike have already been addressed earlier in this chapter. At private universities, as I have noted throughout this book, mission is at the center of everything and living the mission is an important aspect for students and faculty alike. At the private university where this author works, undergraduate students must have a cultural course or experience as part of the core curriculum. This could include studying abroad or participating in a global trip (it could also include taking two semesters of a foreign language). The SON offers several electives that count for meeting the cultural requirement. These courses range from participating in migrant health camps in Mexico to working with orphans and those infected with HIV in Costa Rica. We have a health component to all of the trips, and we have included a mission-fit component.

As part of our graduate curriculum, we have a requirement for a cultural experience. That was one thing that set us apart from other programs and often students chose our master's program because they wanted to have the opportunity to travel abroad, which was one of the ways they could meet that cultural requirement. We had nurse practitioner students traveling with faculty to Mexico, India, and Africa, providing care in remote villages for people who had no other health

Box 10.1 Recommendations Regarding Innovation

- Take chances: You do not know whether something will or will not work unless you try it.
- Try things on a smaller scale first (small tests of change) so that lack of success will not be so detrimental.
- Surround yourself with the right mix of thinkers and doers.
- Change is invigorating.
- Change gets you noticed.
- Do not be satisfied with the status quo: Eventually the status quo becomes outdated.
- Do not be afraid of failure: It is better to have tried and failed then to never have tried at all.
- Small risks can reap high rewards, personally and professionally.
- Nursing education must keep up with the changes in healthcare or students will not be prepared for the practice environments they will face.
- Be open to all ideas: Listen actively.

services throughout the year. But the guidelines for meeting the cultural requirement were very loosely defined and we had some faculty who did not infuse the academic rigor expected for a graduate-level course. One of the first things I worked on with program directors was to tighten the guidelines and develop policies and procedures that were academically and ethically sound. A three-credit global trip had to have three credits worth of educational experiences.

Although many students wanted to travel abroad, it was financially difficult for many and it was also difficult for some to travel and leave families, jobs, and other responsibilities behind for a week to 10 days. So another alternative we developed was a three-credit cultural diversity course that met the culture requirement in the graduate program, but did not require students to travel. Therefore, students had an option to take a global course, or to take an online course that allowed them to gain cultural competence relative to their own communities. We continue to look for opportunities for alternative ways and offerings for which to meet that culture requirement.

Our policies and procedures guiding global travel and the culture requirement were being developed at the same time our university was allocating more human and capital resources to a centralized SA office rather than having individual faculty take responsibility for each of the trips. Part of the strategic priorities for a centralized SA office was to more formally extend and live our mission in sites around the world. This led to university policies and procedures designed to ensure students were safe, the educational experiences were sound, and the cost of studying abroad was overseen in a more stringent manner.

As noted earlier, students must pay for the credits, as well as for the costs associated with the trips. Students' fees for the trip include a portion that covers the faculty members' expenses. Therefore, faculty take the trip for free, even though the expectations for faculty leading global trips are immense. One aspect of the new policies that I initiated was to open up leading global trips to all faculty, not just to the select few who had been leading trips previously. I also discovered that one faculty member was teaching only one class each semester and was then filling her teaching load with global trips, meaning she was out of the country three or four times a year, sometimes with as few as four or five students on a trip. Along with the SA office, we developed policies identifying the minimum number of students necessary to run a global trip (10 students). We also allow only one faculty member to travel with each 10 students, unless a new faculty member is orienting to the trip. We only impose fees for the students to cover the costs of one faculty member for each 10 students, so it does not get too expensive for the students.

Because taking global trips is not "required" as part of our curriculum, either in the undergraduate or graduate programs, as students can meet the culture requirement in other ways, I only award credits toward the teaching load as overload for global travel. Because cultural experiences are a very important part of our mission, I may revisit this policy in the future to determine what is equitable to all faculty.

Our university is an alcohol-free campus, and our SA policies extend that alcohol-free policy to global travel, both for students and faculty. If students or faculty violate that policy, they are subject to the same sanctions as if they violate the policy on campus.

Overall, cultural immersion experiences and global travel are life changing for students and faculty. Policies and procedures should support these rich experiences while at the same time ensuring that there is academic rigor and proper oversight to provide a high-quality learning experience.

REFERENCES

Buller, J. (2014). *Change leadership in higher education*. San Francisco, CA: Jossey-Bass.

Cannella, B., & Finkelstein, S. (2008). *Strategic leadership: Theory and research on executives, top management teams, and boards*. New York, NY: Oxford University Press.

Cowling, W., & Groenwald, S. (2017). Don't judge a nursing college by the way it files its tax return. *Journal of Nursing Education, 56*(5), 255–256.

Fethke, G., & Policano, A. (2012). *Public no more*. Stanford, CA: Stanford University Press.

Hoffman, B. G. (2017). *Red teaming*. New York, NY: Crown Business.

Prather, C. (2010). *The manager's guide to fostering innovation and creativity in teams*. New York, NY: McGraw-Hill.

Ruch, R. (2001). *Higher Ed, Inc.: The rise of the for-profit university*. Baltimore, MD: The Johns Hopkins University Press.

CONCLUSION

We conclude this book with some final thoughts and reflections.

What is your vision for the future of nursing academe in:

Public Universities?

Dr. Neal-Boylan: I would like to see schools of nursing flourish in public universities. Across the country, there is a palpable change in the perception of the value of higher education and decreasing public support for financing public institutions of higher learning. Budget cuts are pervasive so that faculty and administrators who are already "doing more with less" are likely to have to cut valuable programs and employees. Some states have frozen or eliminated tuition. At the same time, public universities are still expected to provide high-quality education. Nurse-run clinics in public universities may cease to exist due to budget cuts. Nursing faculty and administrators will need to become more conversant and comfortable with regard to fund-raising. It may become harder to attract high-quality faculty (and students) to public university programs due to lower salaries and benefits. I hope to see nursing programs not only hang on, but flourish. SON in public universities frequently bring in more students than do other programs in the university. It will be increasingly important for nursing faculty and administrators to advocate for our colleagues in the humanities and sciences who may not bring in as many students but without whom we cannot educate our students.

For-Profit Universities?

Dr. Guillett: I would like to see a real shift in focus from operations to academics. Operations teams should support academics, not drive it. On a larger scale, I would like all schools and clinical partners to break down their silos and work together for the good of the student. Imagine if we trusted each other enough to believe that fundamental skills taught at my school are most likely similar enough to yours that transfer credit could be granted. Think how wonderful it would be if I could call a competing school and have a conversation about sharing a clinical experience to maximize efficiency. We need to standardize nursing education and expand our boundaries.

Private Universities?

Dr. Chappy: I would like to see nursing education and its curriculum be much more fluid and responsive to immediate and future societal trends than to assure NCLEX® pass rates are high. I realize there has to be a test of minimal competence to practice nursing, but I would say that 99.9% of baccalaureate-prepared nurses who graduate from an accredited program are much more than "minimally competent" based on their academic performance while in school. We need to have more clinical rotations in communities, homes, and transitional settings and less in acute care facilities. After all, the majority of nursing care will be delivered outside of acute care facilities in the future and we need to prepare our students for that reality. We need more nurses in schools to ensure children are healthy so they can learn. We need every nurse to be a change agent and a leader. Leaders at private universities can often make curricular changes more quickly than their public-university counterparts. I would like to see private university nursing leaders lead the way in curricular innovation.

What are additional resources you recommend to assist faculty and prospective or current nurse academic leaders in:

Public Universities?

Dr. Neal-Boylan: It is important to keep up with what is going on in the state in which the public university resides. Changes in legislation at the state level frequently impact higher education. I have found *The Chronicle of Higher Education* to be an invaluable resource. Fethke and Policano's *Public No More* (2012) is an interesting and enlightening read. Other sources may also be useful when considering academic leadership roles, in general. Jeffrey L. Buller writes a lot about higher education for faculty and leaders. I have particularly benefited from *The Essential Academic Dean* (2015), *Change Leadership in Higher Education* (2014), and *Positive Academic Leadership in Higher Education: How to Stop Putting Out Fires and Start Making a Difference* (2013). I think books on leadership and leading innovation are also very helpful, such as *The Powell Principles* (2004) by Oren Harari and *Red Teaming* (2017) by Bryce G. Hoffman.

For-Profit Universities?

Dr. Guillett: In addition to the material listed, references that relate to management and leadership skills in general will be of benefit. *Drive* by Pink, *The First 90 Days* by Watkins, and *The 5 Languages of Appreciation in the Workplace* by Chapman and White are good reads and helpful in both navigating and creating the culture. If you are new to the sector, *Higher Ed Inc: The Rise of the For-Profit University* by Ruch is very informative. Keep in mind that laws and regulations regarding the sector are changing and often do so at the mercy of the political environment, so it is best to check the government websites related to for-profit education annually.

Private Universities?

Dr. Chappy: Although these are not specific to private universities, some titles that I found to be excellent resources include *What Got You Here Won't Get You There: How Successful People Become Even More Successful* by Goldsmith (2007); *In Search of Excellence: Lessons From America's Best-Run Companies* by Thomas Peters and Robert H. Waterman, Jr (2012); *Crucial Conversations: Tools for Talking When Stakes Are High* by Kerry Patterson, Joseph Grenny, Ron McMillan, and Al Switzler (2012); *The Five Dysfunctions of a Team: A Leadership Fable* by Patrick Lencioni (2002); *Death by Meeting: A Leadership Fable . . . About Solving the Most Painful Problem in Business* by Patrick Lencioni (2004); and *Good to Great: Why Some Companies Make the Leap and Others Don't* by Jim Collins (2001).

If you had to do it over again, would you work for a (and explain why/ why not):

Public University?

Dr. Neal-Boylan: Yes, I would work for a public university again; however, I would ask many more questions than I did when I first sought to become a chair or dean at a public institution. I have included those questions in the public-university sections of this book. I would also carefully consider the state government and its views on public education, whether or not the majority of the state's legislators are college educated and value public higher education and learning for learning's sake and not just for employment, and the history of financing of public institutions within the state.

For-Profit University?

Dr. Guillett: Yes, I truly enjoy the flat decision-making structure that allows me to have influence over the program and how it is delivered and to know the students individually. I would only work at an institution that had regional accreditation. Nursing students are disadvantaged by national accreditation as it limits credits that can be transferred and in some cases opportunities for graduate school. I also would look carefully at the enrollment goals and retention rates. Schools that are struggling to meet the budget will typically cut academics, which will make the job (whether faculty or leader) exceedingly difficult.

Private University?

Dr. Chappy: Yes, I absolutely would work for a private university again if the mission and values of the organization aligned with mine. Although private schools have to work harder to remain relevant so that students and their families find value in paying the higher tuition required to attend, they have more freedom to change and they lack the political influence to which public universities are subjected. The ability to be more nimble in responding to change at private universities is wonderful. Those who have strong religious convictions and find the ability to live and teach those beliefs infused within the curriculum at a faith-based private school can be truly uplifting. Praying with students and teaching students to pray with patients can create strong bonds and emotional connections that may be missing within public organizations.

What have you learned during your tenure as dean that you would like to share that did not fit into one of the chapters in the book?

Dr. Neal-Boylan: I have learned that the role of academic leader can be extremely rewarding. In addition to developing students, faculty, and staff, one gets to see how all of the intricate pieces of the university puzzle fit (or do not fit) together. However, academic leadership is not for the faint of heart. It is vital to have a good support system of colleagues and friends on whom you can rely for advice, consolation, and just to listen. Nursing is like no other profession and this is nowhere as obvious as in the academic environment. Be prepared for anything and enjoy working with colleagues from other disciplines who can broaden your perspectives in remarkable ways.

Dr. Guillett: Guiding the development and direction of nursing education is one of the most rewarding endeavors a person can undertake. While it demands decisiveness and confidence, it has taught me patience and humility. I am constantly challenged to communicate effectively, and to check and recheck my assessment of the culture and environment. Never underestimate the importance of emotional intelligence in accomplishing your goals.

Dr. Chappy: I am pretty sure that the most important lessons I have learned have been included in at least one chapter of this book. I looked over my "new dean notes" and find all have been addressed. I simply cannot say enough that when you start a new role as dean, you begin as a novice; your faculty expertise remains, but there is so much more to learn. Dr. Neal-Boylan has stressed repeatedly that faculty think they know a lot about what a dean does, but they do not know everything. The "view from the top" is different than the view of the dean role to which faculty have been privy. We desperately need young faculty to strive for and prepare for leadership roles. The demographics of our nursing profession demand it. We need seasoned nurse leaders to share their knowledge and to encourage and support young faculty in moving up in the ranks. I hope that all who read this book are encouraged to advance professionally. Being able to influence the profession is a truly rewarding and fulfilling experience.

REFERENCES

Buller, J. (2013). *Positive academic leadership: How to stop putting out fires ad start making a difference.* San Francisco, CA: Jossey-Bass.

Buller, J. (2014). *Change leadership in higher education.* San Francisco, CA: Jossey-Bass.

Buller, J. (2015). *The essential academic dean* (2nd ed.). San Francisco, CA: Jossey-Bass.

Chapman, G., & White, P. (2012). *The 5 languages of appreciation in the workplace: Empowering organizations by encouraging people.* Chicago, IL: Northfield Publishing.

Collins, J. (2001). *Good to great: Why some companies make the leap and others don't.* New York, NY: Harper Business.

Fethke, G., & Policano, A. (2012). *Public no more.* Stanford, CA: Stanford University Press.

Goldsmith, M. (2007). *What got you here won't get you there: How successful people become even more successful.* New York, NY: Hyperion.

Harari, O. (2004). *The Powell principles.* New York, NY: McGraw-Hill.

Hoffman, B. G. (2017). *Red teaming.* New York, NY: Crown Business.

Lencioni, P. (2002). *The five dysfunctions of a team: A leadership fable.* San Francisco, CA: Jossey-Bass.

Lencioni, P. (2004). *Death by meeting: A leadership fable . . . about solving the most painful problem in business.* San Francisco, CA: Jossey-Bass.

Patterson, K., Grenny, J., MacMillan, R., & Switzer, A. (2012). *Crucial conversations: Tools for talking when stakes are high* (2nd ed.). New York, NY: McGraw-Hill.

Peters, T. J., & Waterman, R. H. (2012). *In search of excellence: Lessons from America's best-run companies.* New York, NY: Harper Collins.

Ruch, R. (2001). *Higher Ed, Inc.: The rise of the for-profit university.* Baltimore, MD: The Johns Hopkins University Press.

Watkins, M. (2013). *The first 90 days: Proven strategies for getting up to speed faster and smarter.* Boston, MA: Harvard Business Review Press.

www.ingramcontent.com/pod-product-compliance
Ingram Content Group UK Ltd.
Pitfield, Milton Keynes, MK11 3LW, UK
UKHW022030300626
6859IPUK00003B/40